Dead Man In My Chair

Alzheimer's Disease Brings Strange Visitors

Carole T. Fulmer

Cee Joy Press
Williamsport, PA

Cee Joy Press

Cover design by If - the Idea Factory, Lock Haven, PA

Library of Congress Control Number: 2007906527

ISBN 978-0-9798957-0-8

ISBN 0-9798957-0-7

First printing - September, 2007

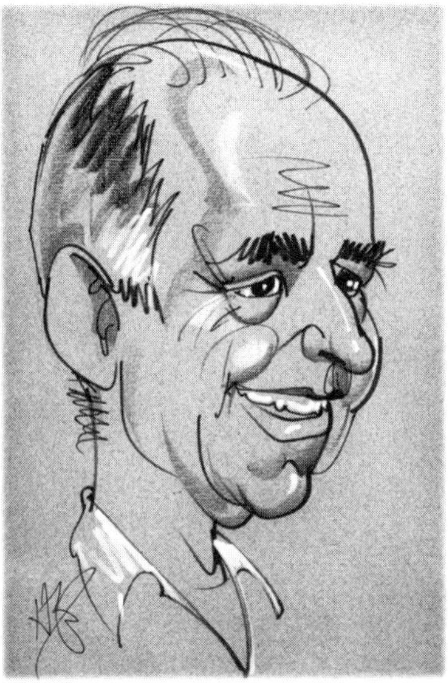

Frank Daniel Fulmer

1924 - 2001

Dedication

In Honor and Memory of
My husband, Frank Daniel Fulmer,
And all those
Affected by dementia or
Alzheimer's disease

Table of Contents

Acknowledgments

It is impossible to thank everyone who brought this book into being, but I do want to mention some special people.

Cecil Murphey, thank you for holding your hand out in faith, and lifting me up when I needed it. I appreciate all your contributions and assistance in publishing this book.

Katherine Yurchak, you showed me that my written stories could be the basis of a book. You planted and nurtured the idea of grouping and publishing these stories. I am grateful for your persistent and ongoing encouragement to bring this book to life.

Thank you Carol Cillo, of If - the Idea Factory, for the artwork.

Pat Shannon, your expertise and editing skills and the midnight hours you freely gave me are of great value.

For all my prayer partners and others who prayed for and supported or had part in creating this book, I give thanks.

Dr. Louise Schaeffer shared my dream of publication. Her writing expertise helped me with *Dead Man In My Chair*. She died before its completion, but her contributions will live on through the book. It was a privilege to work with her.

About the Author

Carole Fulmer has had more than fifty years experience dealing with a loved one with Alzheimer's disease or dementia.

She has been a volunteer for numerous service organizations and devotes many hours each week in service to others. She has worked within the church and healthcare communities.

For more than twenty years she has worked with families dealing with the illness, and continues to grow in her understanding of Alzheimer's disease.

A Word About Henry

Henry is a fictitious character with a fictitious family, acting to bring to life the actual antics of someone with Alzheimer's disease or dementia. The stories demonstrate ways to maximize the good in a variety of situations.

Henry demonstrates the events that actually occurred within my circle of family and friends who had the illness. Through prayers and responses, solutions are displayed. The struggles he models will continue to happen in homes around the world, until a cure is discovered.

Introduction

By Cecil Murphey

"Henry has been acting 'funny.' The doctor calls it dementia, but I call it difficult. I never know what to do..."

Those words express so well the dilemma of the caregiver of persons with dementia. They have no training, no guidebook, and no medical text to explain what they are to do when certain forms of behavior develop.

To make it more complicated, all dementia patients respond differently and there are no guidelines to tell us they're in stage two or five. To make it worse, there is usually little outward change. A close look says that the eyes lose their luster or the gait may be a little slower.

Statistics say that nearly five million people will be diagnosed this year with Alzheimer's or some other permanent memory impairment disease. They don't get better or recover, and no one can stop the progress. The brain cells die and can't be resuscitated.

The disease doesn't kill them and dementia itself doesn't cause physical pain. "He looks so healthy," is something caregivers hear regularly as if to say, "Obviously he's not sick."

But then, as Carole Fulmer points out, they don't have to live with the afflicted person. As she writes about her years of caring for her husband, Henry, she avoids the pitfall of poor-little-me even though she speaks of her discouragement and hardship. At one place she writes, "I learned that I must bend when reality collides with Henry's perceptions. I also learned that in the height of action, it is hard to process the right responses." She stumbled around, she made decisions that didn't prove to be helpful, but she learned.

Now she shares her insights with us. This is a book of Carole Fulmer's personal experiences as she ventured further into her husband's darkness, called Alzheimer's. Although everyone who loves and stands by someone with dementia won't have the same experience, we learn about embarrassment, trying to explain or cover up, frustration, and guilt. Yes, a lot of guilt, as if we could do more. No matter how much we do, there always seems to be more left undone. Despite her inner pain, Carole was able to find humor in many of the situations.

Not only has Carole coped with her husband's debilitating illness but she also has suffered by her friends' attitudes. They no longer visited. Some used the excuse, "I want to remember him the way he was."

Carole also wanted to remember the way he was, but she had to live with him in the present. It wasn't easy when friends disappeared. She often stood alone and watched Henry's day-to-day disintegration. She did find a support group, which helped her cope. She cried with others and they offered their shoulders for her.

Caring for someone with Alzheimer's is difficult, the struggle is long, and discouragement strikes often. As you read this book, you'll realize that you're not alone. Millions of others know and understand your pain, loneliness, and your sense of loss. Carole is only one of them but, thank God, she is one who cares and reaches out.

—Cecil Murphey has written or co-written more than 100 books including 90 Minutes in Heaven and Heaven Is Real with Don Piper. He was a pastor for fourteen years and during most of that time volunteered as a chaplain at local hospitals. He has written several books from a pastor's heart, including When Someone You Love Has Alzheimer's.

Section I
Early Stage

Mysterious Ketchup Bottle

Henry had dementia. It took me a long time to understand. For at least a year I thought something was wrong with me. As I ponder the beginnings of my awareness, I would have to say it started with the ketchup bottle.

To some, things might seem easy to explain; but to me they were not. I thought: *What is going on anyway? I know I threw that empty ketchup bottle away, but since I found it "standing on alert" in the refrigerator, I must have been distracted when I thought I threw it away. I will have to pay more attention to what I am doing and throw it in the trash again.*

Twenty-four hours had flown by since I was last in the refrigerator, then I was staring at a bottle with just a slight painting of ketchup in the bottom. It looked exactly like the one I thought I threw away twice. I started talking to myself: "You're losing it lady. It was bad enough that you thought you threw it away once and you didn't, but now within 24 hours you think you did something and you still didn't do it. Wait a minute! Could Henry have put it back?"

"Nah, I don't think he would be concerned about such things. But before I do anything else, this time I will take it all the way out and make sure it gets into the garbage can."

Throughout the day my mind was drawn to that ketchup bottle and then to the little things that seemed to be wacky at our house. For instance, it seemed as if we spent half the time hunting for lost objects, only to find them in some weird place where I never would have thought to look. Something was wrong, but my mind was not ready to accept just what that was.

It was time for dinner. As I opened the refrigerator door, I could not believe my eyes. It was back again. This time I was going to get to the bottom of the walking ketchup bottle.

"Henry, do you know anything about this ketchup bottle?"

His instant response was, "What about it?" Then he said, "Yeah, I know I have to keep putting it away, because someone keeps throwing it out. You should be more careful."

At first, I felt relief that I was not losing my senses, but then the implications of the fact that my dear sweet Henry was doing it, began to distress me more.

Prayer: - God of the Universe, what's happening? It's only a ketchup bottle. Why am I so upset? I now know that Henry is doing these weird things. God, why? What's going on? Why does he hide things, or retrieve junk from the garbage?

I guess we should check with the doctor, but I don't like to approach Henry with that idea, because of the way he claims there is nothing wrong. He prides himself on never being sick or never needing medical care. Pave the way to get him the help we both need. Direct our paths and keep us safe in your care and comfort. Help us to leave it to you and then take what actions we should. Amen

The Banker

"I'll be a little late getting home," Henry shouted as he rushed for work. "I have to stop at the bank. Payday you know."

"Don't forget to take out the tithe," I called as he whizzed out the door.

Henry seemed so distracted lately. Could he have difficulty with the banking, or is it just my perception?

The day left little time to think of Henry's plans. Too soon, the door burst open with a distraught and disheveled Henry bursting into sight. "I can't do it," he said. "I can't get it right. I have been to the bank five times and I can't get it right."

Before I could respond, he turned and left shouting, "I am going back now before I forget what I want. And don't you dare interrupt me." I was transfixed by this whole outburst.

After he left, the insistently ringing telephone penetrated my consciousness. "The bank,...Yes, my husband was there... He left what? Yes, we'll be glad to get the money... Yes, Henry seems to get confused. Thank you."

What could be wrong with Henry? At first I thought I was imagining things, but I think we need to get a check-up and see if there is a reason for his confusion.

Prayer: - Oh, my Heavenly Father, I don't know where else to turn, but I guess I should have turned it over to you before.

We are concerned about the things that keep happening. Henry has trouble figuring the simplest of tasks. I can't imagine how he could make six trips for a simple deposit and check cashing, then top it off with leaving the money at the bank.

God, please show us the way to go. What should we do? We are frightened. Stay with us and lead us. Amen

Ingredients For Stew

A good stew is made by allowing an assortment of meat and vegetables to cook in their natural juices.

Or, we are said to be "in a stew," when we worry about something, or get into trouble. We are then perceived as "cooking ourselves in our own juices."

Every home is filled with ingredients for stew. But a home where there is illness has a better start, at least for the second kind of stew.

In such a home, it is easy for family members to find some way to place themselves in the broth. It might be about the person who is ill, or about the ability to provide care for the ill person. The natural shifting of roles that occurs when illness strikes is a stew base. Who will be the caretaker, or how that care will be accomplished, can affect the quality of the brew.

The lack, or perceived lack of understanding by family members and others is an ingredient that is not always welcomed. Those not involved in the immediate care frequently lack understanding of how the demands of the situation really play out. That provides vinegar for the broth. Too few hours in the day to accomplish what needs to be done is an ongoing piece of the whole. The finances (or lack thereof) are easy prey for the meat. The ability to produce a safe environment for the ill person also is food for the stew.

Will you choose to make a stew that is edible? Or will you place yourself right in the middle of the kettle?

Our family is trying to make decent stew by eliminating all the destructive ingredients. We strive to work together for the best interest of all--especially Henry.

Prayer: - Most gracious Master, you are well aware of how easily I can get myself right in the middle of the stew. Only you can save me from myself. I fret about the things that may never happen. I borrow tomorrow's troubles. I need the strength to take one day at a time, and leave you in charge of everything.

Your presence is a comfort. When I forget, remind me of that and strengthen us both. Amen

Who's The Boss?

Before illness hit our house, that question was never asked. We always shared responsibilities and the leadership of the family. We were the "boss" of our own domain.

The earth shook and the world vibrated. Big changes rocked us. First, meetings were skipped. Then money was missing. Blank looks replaced Henry's usual confident stance. Questions hung heavy in the air. Excuses were slim or non-existent. Standard answers for any choices were, "I'll do what you do." Or, "I'll have what you have." He seemed incapable of making decisions. Cryptic notes appeared everywhere. Anxiety replaced my husband's easygoing manner.

We weren't quite sure what was happening. But after a lot of battles to get a diagnosis, and much testing, it was decided that dementia (probably the Alzheimer's variety,) was the source of Henry's trouble.

As the disease progressed, one person had to take responsibility for both of us. It was a choice born of necessity and most unwelcome by both of us. Every time we had a disagreement, safety had to prevail. It was not always the happiest of times. Yet, we were soon able to get into a routine and manage.

Prayer: - When I married Henry, there was no question of who was the boss. You were the head of our household and we were a team. We worked together and agreed to share responsibilities. We thought only of "in health and happily ever after" stuff.

Now, teamwork is gone and I must be in charge. Sometimes having responsibility for all this "decision-making" overwhelms me, God. It's tough to choose for myself, but I feel so poorly prepared to decide things for Henry. Lead me to the confidence to choose, and grant me discernment about my choices. Amen

Mysterious Visitors

When I brushed my teeth this morning, I found that those mysterious visitors had come back. You see, Somebody lost the top of the toothpaste tube. I checked around and discovered that Somebody was accompanied by Nobody. (At least, that's what Everybody told me.)

I was about to have some milk for breakfast, but it was warm and sour. Somebody left the carton on the counter. But an investigation proved Nobody was the culprit.

Well, I thought, the least I can do is begin my day with a nice cold glass of juice. But as I lifted the container, it was obvious that Somebody had gotten there before me. The carton was empty. At our house, it seems, Somebody usually comes with Nobody.

Later, when I reached for my footgear, I could find only one black and one brown shoe. "Help," I cried. Of course, Nobody had them. Somebody, however, had seen another pair just like my mismatched shoes somewhere.

I'm off to work now. I reach for my coat. Alas, Somebody took it! Does Anybody know where it is? And do you suppose I can convince Everybody that two different colored shoes are the style?

Prayer: - I guess you can tell that I have to have some humor about all these "body's," around our house. God, I am so thankful for the ability to laugh, otherwise I probably would be crying a lot.

Everyone maintains innocence when something goes wrong. Allow us the freedom to assume ownership of our shortcomings, and help us to forgive the shortfall of others.

Help us to find humor when that would be helpful. Direct our choices. Amen

What You See

I was brought up with the concept: What you see is what you get. My mind focused on what I thought I saw. But that prevented me from seeing things as they really were. Sometimes trusting my observations creates big problems.

Dementia causes serious misconceptions. This is especially true when people don't spend long periods of time with an impaired individual. People who have only occasional encounters with the one suffering with dementia often miss the "tell-tale" signs of this serious illness.

When a family member seeks professional advice, it's sometimes suggested that they're the one who needs help because they are, "too emotionally involved." Explaining the disruption dementia causes in the household, to someone who is unsympathetic, can be a daunting experience.

When our family became concerned about Henry's strange behavior, we feared for his safety. It took a lot of persuasion before Henry agreed to be examined by a physician.

We carried a list of symptoms to the doctor: Henry was usually confused; he drove his car in an unsafe manner; he'd park his car, hitch a ride, and end up far away from home. Then he'd have no idea where he'd left the car. Henry often got lost. Still, Henry insisted on driving his car.

Life with Henry became increasingly difficult. He would put the milk in the closet and the cereal in the refrigerator. He wasn't eating properly. His health was generally deteriorating.

Sometimes Henry was able to function properly, but that usually lasted for short periods of time. Strangers seemed to bring out his best.

When we were with the doctor, I expected to be reinforced in my desire to restrict some of Henry's unsafe practices. But -- wouldn't you know it -- the dementia did not show itself while we were in the doctor's presence.

I tried and tried to explain how badly Henry was functioning on a day-to-day basis, but I tried too hard. So my voice rose up a couple of octaves. And then I was perceived as being "too emotional."

Henry, with all his dementia symptoms, was considered to be the one who was well.

We were told "Henry is fine ... he should be able to manage his daily life without supervision." The doctor even said, "Henry, you can continue to drive your car!" and he turned to me and said, "We have to witness poor driving before we can make judgements about taking a license."

As I said, what you see is not what you get. Sometimes trusting our observations can create big problems.

Prayer: - Lord, sometimes people believe what is not true. Surround us with those who seek the truth and with people who are sensitive to others. Cause Henry's daily behaviors to become evident to those who need to make judgments about his care. Lead those who criticize me to spend enough time with him so as to realize that he has short bursts of lucidity. Lord, we need patience and understanding, not criticism. Grant us peace. Amen

The Chicken Is On The Counter

The day started like any other. I had some chores to do in town, so I placed a package of frozen chicken out to thaw and went about my business. My husband happily "puttered around" the house. I felt secure in leaving him alone.

When I returned with my tasks completed, I raced to prepare dinner. I couldn't find the chicken. It wasn't where I thought I left it. I decided not to panic, but to pause and review what I'd done with it. I retraced my steps, but still could not find it. I tried to think. Where could it have gone? It isn't where it should be. Now, I even question my ability to recall. Henry is the only person here. I can't think of anything more reasonable.

"Henry, do you know what happened to my chicken," I questioned.

His response was hard to believe, so I queried, "You put the chicken where?"

He responded again, "I buried it!"

When I recovered enough to speak, I squeaked, "Why would you do that?"

He immediately responded, "The chicken was as hard as a rock, and I knew it was petrified."

I had to admit that it was hard as a rock. I also realized that if you couldn't remember about freezing foods, you would believe it was ready for the dump. I did find the humor in this illogical logic.

When I paused to think, I appreciated that he was able to string information together. Still, I wished that he could use all the available truths and come to a more workable conclusion. I wanted my chicken!

The humor in Henry's mismatched logic could not put chicken on the table, but it did remind me that I need to be clear in speaking about what is happening. I must assume nothing, and therefore explain everything.

Prayer: - God, it's me again. I thought things were under control. But then Henry buried the chicken. Forgive me for getting so excited when it happened. I am ashamed of myself because I was yelling at Henry when he told me what he did. Then, it did strike me funny, and

I could follow his confused thinking. If I knew nothing about frozen food, I might behave in the same way. Now I know he really was aiming to make things easier. I thank you for allowing me to see the humorous side, and that he was trying to assist as well.

It would be helpful to both of us if I could see these trouble areas before they happen. God, lead us to ways to prevent such misunderstandings from transpiring. I will be most appreciative. I need your direction and support. My sense of humor has saved the day here. Help us to cultivate the ability to enjoy the comic side of life. It makes the days pass more comfortably and more easily.

Thank you for all your gifts. Amen

Divided Load

I am often overpowered by the weight of the responsibility as caregiver for my husband, Henry, who has dementia. I crave help from my family.

Alice, my sister said, "I am perfectly willing to do anything to help you."

That wasn't working, so I asked Alice, "What is the exact meaning of what you are offering?"

Alice exclaimed, "I am willing to come over any time you want me to, and to do whatever you want me to do."

I reluctantly said, "Your answer makes me feel as if I am begging, and I don't like that. I would like you to volunteer to offer specific choices and times. For instance, I would like you to say: 'I am available Monday, Tuesday, Thursday. . . or whatever days you are available.' Then I want you to say, 'I will take Henry;' or 'I will do a certain task;' or 'I can make it possible for you to do something like mow the lawn, . . . etc., etc."

The difficulty is that I had very clear ideas about what I wanted Alice to do, but I was afraid to hurt her feelings by actually stating my own needs. I feel guilty for needing help. I simmered with anger because I felt misunderstood and unsupported.

The reality was that when Alice was given the understanding and the opportunity, she freely offered what I needed. It was hard to find a way to be totally honest with her . . . to spell it out. I told her, "I feel there is something wrong with me, because I need someone to relieve me of taking care of Henry."

I told Alice the things that make me feel bad about getting help. When I did, the weight lifted. My anger was dissipated. For the first time since Henry became ill, my sister and I clearly and openly communicated. It was the beginning of a new and happier family relationship.

Prayer: - I was mad at the world, God. I felt that no one was listening to me . . . including you. You know how overwhelmed I was. When Alice started talking, it seemed so natural to speak up. Thank you for providing a way for us to jar the door to engage in open and honest communication. I wasn't aware of the anger that I was carrying. I know I also had trouble talking to you at those times. Forgive me.

I know you promised to carry our burdens, but that felt more meaningful today, as I realized that my anger was keeping me from you.

This whole experience has helped me interact with Sis as well. I suspect that I am the one who changed, because I feel more peaceful. That is obvious in Henry's actions as well. It is a joy to witness the differences as they filter through.

Cause your love to trickle into all of us and strengthen us to work together in unity and peace. We continue to sing your praises. Amen

Free As A Bird

In the warmth of the afternoon, I was busily engaged in preparing dinner. I never heard the whispered opening and closing of the door. Silence reigned. I thought that I had better investigate what was happening, because Henry was prone to leave and wander off somewhere because of his dementia. Silence could mean trouble. I looked, and then I called. There was no Henry! But what was that in the corner of the room?

As I went to investigate, the urgent ring of the telephone beckoned. The caller explained why that pile was in the corner. It was Henry's clothing. He had wandered, naked to my lady friend's home. She was distraught and begged me, "Do something, and do it right now."

With a red face and Henry's clothing, I rushed to her home. Henry seemed content and undisturbed about the situation. In fact, he was laughing and joking. His explanation that: "I was hot, so I decided to go for a walk." That didn't diminish my need to get him clothed. The neighbor was "rattled" as well.

Henry had difficulty understanding why I was fussing, and I surely was doing my share of that. He explained, "I don't know what the big deal is. I was hot, and my clothes were sweaty. I took them off. Why do you make an issue about it?" Since he had no discomfort walking down the street naked, I didn't know where to begin. But I tried. I was able to convince him that for today, clothing was the way to go.

Shaking, after a struggle getting him dressed, I offered an apology and thanks to our neighbor, and then took Henry home. He was unhappy, but I was relieved.

I had to re-think my supervision of his care, and watch him more closely. In a short time, in high and low places, I installed latches and alarms on the doors. I am more vigilant about silence, but I still fear a rerun of this episode.

Prayer: - I was a wreck today, God. It was hard for me to hold it together. It happened so quickly that I didn't know what to do. I often react with the situation. I forget to call on you. Then I find myself more impatient, or more upset. Help us both to be sensitive to your constant presence, particularly in such stressful situations.

I know that if Henry were well, he would have been humiliated by doing something so different from our values. As it stands, I feel enough embarrassment for both of us. If you could protect Henry from his actions, I would be most appreciative. Allow him a sense of freedom, yet protection. It's so difficult to draw the line at the right place.

As the rain refreshes, allow this storm to refresh us and move us forward in the sense of your presence. Guide us in all we say and do. Amen

Positive Reinforcement

Am I able to accept the challenge to make a difference for Henry and his impairment because of dementia? I have done it before. My plan is simple. First, I need to step back from the issues of dealing with my love with a disease, and then evaluate how I would feel if I were in his situation. What clues has he given me concerning his perspective about where he is, and what is happening to him?

I absorbed his anguish; then I worked on giving him guidance. We planned activities with tasks that were easy to accomplish. He can do many of the minor household tasks, if he is given enough instructions. Finishing a project instilled in him a sense of accomplishment. But it is a challenge to find chores within his realm of ability. Yet, his pride is worth the effort.

I praise him more freely for what he can do, because it makes us both feel good. I know that we all can stand recognition.

Prayer: - Thank you for the reminders to affirm my Henry. He struggles to do his best. His best today is not even his worst of years ago, yet I am filled with thanksgiving for what we do have. The losses seem to fill me with more of an appreciation of each day.

Father, I ask that this robber of the mind be taken away from him and that he be restored to health. But thy will be done. I know that you have promised that you are with us for the journey. For that, we give thanks. Amen

The Wilted "Tassel"

My city upbringing has given me a great appreciation for the opportunity to grow my own food. Although our garden was small, we grew all sorts of vegetables.

Henry joined the ritual of weeding and checking the day's growth in the garden.

I had never seen carrots growing before. In the store, they have the tops removed, so I didn't know much about them. Henry said the lacy tops were the "tassel."

Everything looked fine, but the carrot "tassels" were wilted. I didn't know why, but my reasoning was that they ought to be watered, and then later checked. Their droopy tops puzzled and concerned me. What was the problem? I was sure that water would help. But later when I looked, they were still droopy. And now they were soggy wet. After several days of nursing them, I said, " "Henry, what do you think is the matter with the carrots?"

In one breath he said, "I have no idea. Each one looked fine when I pulled it out to check on it."

Prayer: - Father, thanks for the answer to the mystery of the wilted "tassel." It is no wonder they wilted. It is funny that Henry is so innocent and that he had no idea that he was ending the life of my carrots. He thought that he was helping me. I'll need to watch him more closely, God. Guide me to anticipate these misinterpretations.

Thank you for our garden and its abundance, and even the lesson about carrots. We have so many other gifts for which to give thanks. We praise you. We worship you. We are filled with overwhelming joy and thanksgiving. Amen

The Aged Bride

The world has gone topsy-turvy since Henry has been acting "funny." The doctor calls it dementia, but I call it difficult. I never know what to do. I let others deal with him when I can.

We were looking at family pictures today and I was unaware that Henry became convinced I was not the same person as his wife in the pictures. He recognized the "me" of my youth. Because I am clothed in a body that is forty years older, he did not know that I was the same person.

Unaware of the change in his thinking, I joined him and headed for bed. He became very nervous, He refused to get undressed in front of me.

I finally realized that he was not aware we were married to each other. I tried to think what I would do if I didn't know we were married. I realized that I wouldn't go to bed with a stranger. Although he knew my name, now I was a stranger. Because he didn't know I was his wife, his behavior was proper.

I decided to allow him to be alone and get ready for bed, and waited until he fell asleep. I then climbed into bed and slept.

The next morning, when he awoke he remembered my identity., "Boy," he said, "I am so glad you came."

I learned that I must bend when reality collides with Henry's perceptions. I also learned that in the height of action, it is hard to process the right responses. I hope this experience will lead me to be more understanding and helpful next time.

Prayer: - Dear Father, I feel so helpless in dealing with Henry. My mind says I should feel and act one way, but I respond in another. I become upset when this happens.

Today, when Henry thought I was not his wife, I wanted to run and hide . . . or to cry. I didn't want to hear it. I felt as if I couldn't handle the situation. I now know that he really was convinced that we were not married. I need strength to be able to remain in this situation and work with my husband while I look for a solution to reach and understand him.

I pray that we both have the strength and wisdom to know what to do and how to react. I also want to know how to keep my emotions in check . . . to find a channel for them . . . or even discover a way to manage them better.

Bless us all and help us to learn from each new experience. Thank you for allowing peace to prevail once again. Amen

Section II
Middle Stage

Pass The Jello, Please!

As we sat down to dinner, our first family get- together in months, chaos reigned. The children were chattering excitedly. As I served the little ones, the people at the table grew silent as Henry grabbed the plate away from one of the girls and took all that was on it. The youngster was upset, but Henry was unaware of that. He proceeded to claim the child's dessert as well. I knew that when he was acting like he was, it would be impossible to reason with him.

All the children were upset. Monica began to cry softly. She was calling "Me-maw," my grandmotherly name. As we met, I smothered her in a hug and listened to her fears. "Why is Pop-Pop acting like that? He took my favorites."

"Monica, Pop-Pop has a sickness that makes him act differently. When he wants something, he can't remember that he could have his own without taking yours. Can you help Me-maw fix your new special plate? I like the way you arrange your food." A few sniffles later, peace was restored.

Oh, the unwelcome change that has come! Henry was always the patient one. The children were his delight. He would turn cartwheels on the lawn for them, and he was always a "soft touch" for whatever they wanted. That is why his behavior creates such emotion and is difficult to handle. It's still a challenge to remember all the precautions I need to take.

I did think that Henry's snack would hold him until I served the girls, but I think he forgot that he had eaten. Next time I will make sure that Henry is separated from the little ones and he has his plate full so that he might be more inclined to leave the children alone.

Prayer: - Father, God, just when I think I have this patience thing under control, Henry comes up with a new caper, and I have to work on it again. I so want to protect the children, but I want to protect Henry as well. I keep forgetting that it is his illness that makes him behave so radically.

Father, you can make the children feel safe and protect them. Help me to take whatever steps are necessary to make it happen. Heighten Henry's awareness and give us all strength. In all things we give thanks. Amen

Strange Bedfellows

I was tired. Although it took a while, Henry climbed into his pajamas on his own. While I finished my final tasks of the day, I heard him clamber into bed.

As I came into the room I was confronted with an all too familiar sight. Henry was in bed, in his "pjs, " and with his baseball cap secured tightly on his head.

I don't know all the reasons why that bothered me so much, but it did. We were always brought up with the idea that it was a sign of disrespect to wear a hat in the house, and it felt strange to me. I thought, *I'm glad nobody can see this one.*

"Henry, we're going to bed. We don't usually wear our hats to bed."

Henry set me straight. He said, "I do. I always do!"

Leaving him in his hat left me feeling as if there was an urgent task to be done. I thought: *Carole, that's your problem. He's happy in his hat and he is not going to be convinced that it is strange.* It was a restless night.

I thought that ours was the only family with this experience until at an Alzheimer's Support Group meeting, someone came in and said, "My dad wears his hat to bed, and it drives me crazy."

Another person spoke up and said, "My husband does that too."

And another said, "Sometimes mine wants to wear regular clothing to bed as well."

I realized that I was not alone with having to deal with this issue. It didn't change anything, but me. We laughed because we had company, but we all felt as if we were the only ones, and strange as well. Most of us wouldn't tell anyone it was happening. It was embarrassing even to mention it in the group.

Knowing others were troubled in the same ways helped me. I said to myself, "Lighten up, Carole, set priorities."

Prayer: - Father, you did it perfectly today, as you so often do. A simple, almost ridiculous thing to be upset about agitated me and you sent me to the right place and to the right people from whom to get the help. The support group helps me to be with people who have been experiencing the same problems and feelings. Sometimes, just knowing that someone else actually is confronted with a similar thing, is all I need to make it easier.

Master, we have so many blessings. Thank you. Help me to keep things in perspective and to be more patient with Henry's new habits. I have a lot to learn. Along the way, allow me to draw strength from you. Amen

Doorway To The World

It was a cool, crisp, sunny day. Before involving myself in the day's activities, I opened the storm door to let in nature's beauty. As I released the door, it slammed shut.

How strange! The door was operating properly when I went through it only hours before. While checking for the problem, I had to reach for the glass panes. Suddenly they dropped to the floor.

Further inspection revealed that the clips and screws that held the panes in place were missing. Also missing were parts of the air device that slowed the door's closing.

"Henry, do you know anything about this door?"

"Yeah," he responded with a grin. "I fixed it for you."

Angry and frustrated, but being careful to take a deep breath, I asked, "Henry, do you know where the screws and clips are?"

"Somebody came and took them all," was Henry's response.

I wanted to blurt out, "And was that somebody wearing your clothes?"

Someday I may locate the place where Henry hides the gadgets he removes when he "fixes things" for me. Meanwhile, I've convinced myself that I don't need to open the storm door. I have enough to do in dealing with Henry's new occupation of trying my patience. He's so good at what he does.

Prayer: - You are the keeper of all, Father. We have a lot of things that are misplaced. Many are objects that we think we need to manage the home. Direct us to their hiding places and keep things from becoming lost. We need patience for both of us. We struggle so much to live patiently. Allow your love to shine through us. Amen

Department, Please!

It was time for me to go grocery shopping. Our adult son, Walter, had come to see that Henry didn't get into any irreparable mischief. Henry was in a restless state, so I was apprehensive about leaving. If Henry really set his mind to do something he shouldn't, I had the notion that Walter would have trouble with his Dad,.

As soon as my car pulled out of the driveway, Henry picked up the telephone to call about our broken hairdryer. He spoke clearly into the phone, "Yes, I'll wait until you transfer me to that department... Yes, I have a broken vacuum cleaner I want to talk about... Yes, I'll wait until you transfer me to that department... Idiots! Yes, I have a broken hairdryer I want to talk about... You want to transfer me to that department? Can't you morons get anything straight?"

For the entire time I was gone, Henry spoke to one department head after the other. He hurled horrible insults, and became more excited with each transfer of the call. When he got the right department, Walter called out "It's a hairdryer, Dad." But that left Henry shouting at Walter as well. Walter could not convince him to call later, nor could he persuade him to say the right thing when he did have the right department. Walter became so excited trying to get his attention and to change what was happening, that he was shouting almost as much as Henry shouted.

When I came, Walter welcomed me as never before. His words tumbled together as he raced to place the events of the morning into my charge. Our six foot two, "take charge son," was worn out and wanted to go home. He was in charge for one hour, and already he had his fill of coping for the day.

Prayer: - We're here, God. My two men have had a rough day. We all need help in dealing with this changed, frustrated Henry. You know that Henry would not behave that way in good health. Help us to remember that.

Guide us to nurture the positive and affirm all we encounter, including ourselves. You have promised that you would provide all our needs. I hope you will agree that we all need big doses of patience and perseverance, and then grant us that.

Some day we will be able to laugh at some of the things that hap-

pen, but today is not the day. If you would shine your light on the lighter side of things, we would be helped.

Keep all of us, but especially Henry, in the capsule of your care. Amen

Devoured By A Sadness

I am devoured by a sadness that goes to the depths of my spirit. The sadness knows no bounds, it is all consuming. It is not proper to speak of it because no one died. Yet, there is a part of him that is forever changed. He is slowly fading from my grasp.

Allowing my feelings makes it difficult to smile. To deny the feelings creates incredible pain and loneliness. To put the pain into words helps, but when no one seems to understand what it means, I feel more alone than before. I want to be held and comforted, but the one I desire for that is unable to understand or respond, and sometimes he doesn't even know who I am. The tears move slowly down my cheeks. I want to scream or pound on every door and say, "Don't you know my love is fading away?" But, I scream inside in silence, because it is what is expected. I protect the others, they have their own troubles.

Somehow, I figure I can get through. I cry out to God, and it seems as though even He is far away. I know I have many blessings. I try to focus on the best of the bad, then things are not quite so bleak. I pray for a living person to talk to. How can that be, when I am unwilling to cast my burdens on another?

I can always see others whose lot is much more difficult than mine. and if given a choice between their troubles and mine, I would take my own. Yet, that does not remove the sadness.

Just when I think I have my sorrows under control, I find that there's another loss or difficult change. Struggling through the tough times, I wonder if I have the strength to keep going.

Those who believe that Henry's illness is some sort of punishment, burden my heart.

I know that he is totally dependent upon my care. I must keep myself well, but my mortality concerns me. What will he do if I'm not around? There's no other as understanding to take the responsibility of his care. I know because I find problems getting someone to fill in for short periods of time. Yes, my sadness has no bounds.

Prayer: - Father, when sadness consumes me, allow me to feel the love you shower on me. I pray for acceptance of your will and your way in all that I do. God forgive me, but sometimes I question if your opinion of my ability to cope is greater than the ability I actually have.

I feel so ill equipped to deal with all the ramifications of this disease, and I fear for the days ahead. Help me to take one day at a time and focus on the things that are positive and nurturing. Allow me to feel your strength and guidance to reach out to those who need my help and love. Show me the way to maximize the ability Henry has, and the best means to support him.

I do worship you. I praise you, and I give thanks to you. Amen

Quick-Change Artist

I had the time perfectly figured out. It always takes Henry 1-1/2 hours to get dressed and 45 minutes to eat a light breakfast, and it would take us 20 minutes to get to the church for the memorial service. Everything was going smoothly. There were only 21 minutes left before the service. Henry was dressed and I was ready to make a last minute powder-room stop, and then leave.

When finished, I figured we had exactly enough time to drive to the church. "Henry where are you?" There was silence. "Henry, answer me!"

He sauntered out of the bedroom in his tee shirt, blue jeans and a baseball cap. He had changed in record time. Now time became my enemy. He could not completely change again. Besides he was insisting, "Everyone wears jeans to funerals."

I managed to get him into a shirt, but there was no way to convince him to change into anything else. He then asked, "What else should I wear besides a baseball cap?"

The cap seemed anchored to his head. I paused to gather my patience, and think it through. I knew that God would excuse whatever he wore, but I wasn't sure my friends would understand. My pride was in my throat, but I decided it was better to be there, "as is," than to stay away. It would be a bonus if they understood, but if they didn't, "so be it." At least, I tried my best.

I held my head high and expressed my love to my friends, and I was grateful that they acted as if nothing was awry. I am thankful for my blessings.

Prayer: - My thoughts are not as important as I like to believe they are. God help me to search out your will and way for me. Help me to keep the way Henry behaves in perspective.

In my effort to make him look his best, it appears I make him unnecessarily uncomfortable. I must admit that he was happier in his choice of slacks and a cap. When I thought that you would probably accept his attire; I was freed to attend to my friend's sorrows.

I now realize that I can be almost as stubborn as Henry is about making changes. Grant me help to be open to the things that I should support, and give me the wisdom to step away from those things that don't matter. Grant me the grace to know the difference. Amen

Reveille!

It was the end of a busy day. Henry was into his blue pajamas and in bed by 11:00 PM. Now I could finish my work. When my tasks were completed, I headed for the bedroom and saw that it was going to be another one of those endless nights. Henry was dressed and shaving. "What are you doing?" I asked.

Smugly he pronounced, "I am getting ready for church."

When I told him it was the middle of the night, he became very upset. I figured I had better let him finish shaving. Maybe his memory would work for us and cause his determination to head for church to diminish. But, it was not meant to be.

He was focused on calling someone to get a ride to church. "I can drive you to church," I told him. That only upset him more.

In exasperation he commanded me, "You'd better stop this silliness. You know you're not old enough to drive."

Deep within, I laughed silently at the absolute absurdity of being mistaken for someone who wasn't old enough to get behind the wheel of a car.

When I collected my composure, I tried to suggest, "Don't you remember we always call for a ride closer to the time we want to leave? It's a bit early to call right now." He backed off then, and agreed to wait.

But within a few minutes, I made another mistake when I suggested that he put on his PJs.

"I'm not getting undressed," he snapped at me. "I'm just going to lie down here for a while and rest my eyes."

So, if you see my husband in church in slightly rumpled clothes that look as if he slept in them, you're probably right.

Now you know why I'm filled with gratitude that Henry is part of a circle of love--that he's in a place where he's found freedom.
We need everyone to be a part of that circle too.

Prayer: - Here I am, Father, with my day before you. The absurdity of Henry believing I was not old enough to drive, lightened the weight of losing my sleep. Henry's illness has helped me to feel years beyond my age. Although nothing changed, I felt younger and my heart was lighter, when he said that.

I am constantly being reminded to select the areas that are worthy of changing or being concerned about. Strengthen me in my choices. Amen

I Fixed It!

Mowing the lawn used to be Henry's job. Now, confused as he was, it had become mine.

It had rained and remained wet for ten days. When I was working with one of my mowers, it kept stalling. As I brought the mower in, Henry wiped his hands on the oily rag. Then with a broad grin he said, "I fixed it for you."

Panic seized me as I asked what he did. He proudly stated that he had, "gassed the mowers."

With trepidation, I asked, "What did you put in them?"

My fears were realized. He'd used a combination of gas and oil in "all the holes." Now I understood why the mower I was using was stalling. He had "fixed" the two mowers. My next stop was the repair shop.

The repairman was unhappy when he saw what happened. When the shop owner returned our mowers, he informed me that the mess was terrible, and that he would not repair the mowers if a similar thing happened again.

The next day, I assumed my machines were ready to work. When I tried the mower again, gasoline splashed out of the carburetor. It would not start. When I tried to find what had happened, I discovered that Henry had filled the tank by spilling gas into the carburetor. He had tried hard to help me, but I still had to wait for the mower to dry out.

On the next day I was served with papers. I would be penalized for having grass over five inches, and would spend fifteen days in jail or pay a $50.00 fine. I had three days to comply, and then any further complaints would bring about the fines or sentencing.

It seemed unreasonable to enforce the law without consideration of the circumstances. I fantasized loaning Henry to the police to see if they could make out as well as I.

Prayer: - Henry was always able to take care of everything. Now he struggles. Ease my impatience, God. I get upset when other people seem eager to complain and yet, they do nothing to help me. Fill our minds with things that we can do to make it easier for each of us.

Henry works to do the things he always did well, but he can't remember how to do them. Oh how we miss those days! Ease our sadness.

Carrying the responsibilities for both of us is difficult. Give me the strength to do what he can't. Amen

Bigfoot

I was busily engaged in housecleaning, when Henry rushed past me with a purposeful stride. Something alerted me to trouble, I was sure things were not as they seemed. "Henry where are you going?"

With a too-happy face he announced, "I am going to the garbage can."

I looked closer and saw that he had all my socks. Hurriedly I requested, "What are you doing with my socks?"

Without a pause he asked, "You mean these big old things? They aren't yours. They are too big for anyone in this house. I am going to throw them out."

I blurted, "I know my feet are big, but those are my socks and I need them." I looked into his eyes and knew that he was unconvinced. I needed to regroup. Okay! "Henry, can you put those aside for a minute and run some things out to the car for me?"

As soon as Henry entered the yard, I hid the socks and manufactured one task after another to keep him occupied. When he stopped running, he forgot about the socks for this time. Judging from the number of things missing, and the things recovered, I had missed some of his trips to the garbage can with my valuables. The other day I discovered that just before pick-up time, he deposited $20.00 worth of new light bulbs as refuse. I didn't discover them until they were gone forever.

I must say that it is never boring around here. He is so-o-o creative and full of things to do.

Prayer: - Master, I am filled with thanks. When I am able to find humor in some of these strange situations in which I find myself, I feel less overpowered.

Henry has a way of cutting me down to size. I know I have big feet, but I still don't think that they are so big that I have to hide my socks. He thought they were big. At least, he told me what he was thinking. Thank you, for that.

I pray for help to keep Henry out of the things that are troubling. If there is a way to think ahead and avert losing useful things, place that way in my mind. Strengthen us both. Amen

Electronic Assault

Henry was up and the day's activities were well in hand. Moving around, my thoughts were invaded by a blaring cacophony. I had to get at its source and stop it now. The noise was grating and very penetrating.

I hustled in the direction of the sound, when Henry called out, "What are you doing?"

I responded, "I am going to shut down the noise."

Instantly, Henry jumped in front of me, and in one breath he said, "This is my radio and I am listening to it and I don't want you to touch it. I have it fixed perfect, and you would only mess it up."

"Henry, could I just tune it to your favorite program and turn it down a little bit?"

He came back sharply with a don't cross me type, "NO!"

I backed off and thought, *Patience, Carole. Think of a different way.*

OK, get the portable radio and tune it in to his show.

"Henry, I have this radio set to your program. You could go to the other room and listen, and I would be out of your way". . .and internally added, *I can shut off that noise and restore a balance.*

It worked! He took the portable and left and with joy, I turned off the other radio. Normal household sounds were restored. Ah-h-h-h, what peace!

Prayer: - Lord, I feel as if I have put in a full day already. Help me to calm myself. You know I dislike having confrontations with Henry. I need to think of the right responses to his changed personality and behaviors. I have to slow down and think without reacting. Lead me to better ways to work things through. Help me to slow down and rest. Without your help, I would be lost. Thank you, Father, and thank you for your patience with me. Amen

The Furnace Repairman

It was an icy, freezing cold night. I felt "warm and toasty" and was happy to be home, ready to fall into bed. It was 1:00 AM and I was exhausted, but still trying to get Henry motivated to get in bed too. "Henry where are you?"

After a period of silence, he answered, "I am watching the water coming out of the furnace I fixed."

"What water? What fixing? Not again! Oh God, please don't let it be what it sounds like!"

When I checked, the furnace had steaming hot water coming from the boiler. At the rate the water was pouring out, I was afraid the basement would be flooded before morning. I knew that it was a "premium service-call" time, for the second time in a week! But I couldn't wait this time, either.

The furnace man was most gracious about being called out of bed on a cold night. Then he took me aside and said, "Lady, there are parts missing. What am I supposed to do? These parts never break down, so I don't have spare ones. I think that we don't even have them in the shop."

I answered, "Let me see if my husband knows where he put them."

I took Henry aside and asked, "Do you know where the furnace parts are?"

He surprised me when he answered, "Yes I do."

I thought, finally he remembers where he put something.

I asked, "Where are they?"

He pulled me off to the side and whispered, "See that furnace man over there, he is not very good, because he took the parts for his collection."

My sweet innocent one firmly believed that he was blameless, and that I had contracted a thief. I had to convince him to keep his thoughts secret, so that he wouldn't insult the furnace repairman.

The worker went out and rummaged in his truck. He returned with the needed parts and said, "I had the whole apparatus in the truck, so I removed the part from that and can now make the repairs."

Prayer: - Father, having to call the repairman in the middle of the night is very upsetting. Henry did finally tell me that we had trouble. Thank you for that. It would have been better, if the furnace was not disabled.

I guess you are telling me that I need more patience, and that's right. My impatience is a handicap and an asset. Allow me to use it for good. Accept my thanks for the furnace. It's a bitter, cold night and we are now warm. Thank you. Amen

The Scallions

It was a glorious day, especially designed for working out of doors. We were headed for what I called my "city garden," (a lot of garden in a small amount of space,) to undertake a much-needed weeding.

As Henry tagged along, I said, "I hope those scallions are ready to eat, because I have been hungering for them."

Henry's response was, "Which are they?"

"You know, what you call spring onions," I shot back.

We reached the patch quickly, and I could not believe what I saw. Every one of the young onions had been trampled down and ground into the earth. "Who-o-o would do this," I gasped.

As I looked up, Henry was smiling broadly and said, "I did."

Softly I said "Why?"

"I wanted to help you."

"Let me get this straight, you wanted to help me? How would that help?"

"I don't know, I just know that was my job in Grandma's garden, and I wanted to help you like I helped her. She used to say it made them grow bigger, so I wanted to get out here as soon as I remembered to make 'em grow for you."

Sensing my upset, Henry came close and said, "I was just trying to make it easier for you."

Calming myself, I took a deep breath and said, "It's OK Henry. Don't worry about it. We can get spring onions at the market."

I said to myself; "Learn the lesson that good intentions don't put scallions on the table, and Carole, "ya gotta" to learn to laugh. He was doing the right thing, he just did it before they grew, and then he killed the whole thing. It's just onions, Carole."

Prayer: - Father I feel so good when I can come to the garden, but today was different. Henry was so proud, and I was so disappointed. I had trouble being very understanding and following through on the good I felt. When I became upset, guilt overwhelmed me. Thank you for inspiring me to ask Henry why he did it, because that eased the situation. When I think about it, it is nice to know that even though he was misdirected, he was thinking of me.

But you can see I still need big doses of patience and understanding. Grant me a sufficient amount of each, according to your will and way. Thank you. Amen

Are You Awake?

Sleep is a scarce commodity at our house. Henry likes to wander around at night. He will fall asleep the minute he sits in a chair. To him, nights are meant for roaming. His little naps are enough to take the edge off his sleep and keep him going indefinitely.

His snoozes don't rest me a bit, but they do provide an opportunity for me to do the things that upset him when he is awake. Exhaustion continues to be my enemy. I crave rest, ah-h-h blessed rest, even a little bit would help.

Henry's softly whistling breathing alerted me to nap time. Maybe if I could sleep when he does, I could find my rest. I'll try a quick one.

I hardly shut my eyes when he stirred. Whoops, he's up already. Soon my name is whispered. "Carole, Carole, Carole, Carole, Carole, Carole." Each one becomes louder than the one before. If I ignore him, will he get quiet and sit back down? Instead, he began calling, "Are you awake?" Finally it became a trumpeted bellow. "Are you awake?"

I waited until he repeated it several times, and then answered, "Yes, what do you want."

Smiling he said, "I just wanted to see if you were sleeping."

Prayer: - Here I am, in the need of prayer. You told me to give thanks in all that I do. Sometimes it is difficult to be truly thankful. Today, I readily give thanks that Henry is able to be up and around. I am especially thankful for that, because each day there is more loss and I don't know how much time he has to be mobile. He is much easier to care for when he is able to navigate alone.

I need rest, God. Show me the things you would have me do, and wash me with your healing balm. Refresh me. Restore me, that I may follow you each step of the way. Amen

My Mask

I wear my mask to hide things I don't want you to see ... my fears, my imperfections, my weaknesses ... things like that. I also hide my helplessness and 'differentness'-- and anything else that has gone awry in my personal world. My disguise protects me in the "now." It's a shield for me as I live with Henry's Alzheimer's disease.

Please understand me, I don't want charity. I'm willing to carry my load. My responsibilities are mine. But I can't bear to have you see the violence of the once mild-mannered love of my life. I hide the pain my husband's changes have brought about. When I mask the reality of how bad things are, they seem better to me. And when I disguise my fears, I feel less afraid.

How strange! Wearing the mask closes doors to the support and understanding I crave. But to remove the mask makes me vulnerable. Then again, maybe if I lift the mask a bit and share some of my thoughts, we both would be more comfortable.

I do need to explain to you how Henry's illness has robbed the man I love of his usual gentle disposition. You need to understand that it's the illness that has brought about these changes. What's happened to him is not the result of a perverted sense of his will.

We're a proud couple--Henry and I. Our vows, "Til death do us part," made us totally committed to each other. Each of us would sacrifice the world for the other. But now our world has tilted way out of control.

Why do I feel this horrible grief? No one has died. Should I dare expose this awful sadness to you, I'd be revealing a pain that never can be comforted. Then again, maybe ... if I drop my mask a bit ... maybe if I told you the truth ... we all would be enriched.

Will you help me let this happen? Will you reach out to me as I drop my mask? No other person in the world should ever have to experience my masked life.

Prayer: - It is easy to hide, even from you, dear heavenly Father. Sometimes I even hide from myself. It is better when we are open and honest in our dealings, but there are many reasons we are not. We try to protect our family and we are afraid to expose our feelings.

We crave acceptance and fear hurting or burdening others.
Show us the proper balance in all that we do.
Guide us each step of the way. Amen

Gun To My Head

We spent this snowy, cold day doing things that wearied me. I was ready for bed, when mild-mannered Henry appeared toting a gun, demanding, "It's time you went home."

Startled, I replied, "But, Henry, I live here."

That was the wrong thing to say, because that only infuriated him. With a reddening face and a much louder voice, he commanded, "You are going to leave now!"

I didn't even know if the gun was loaded, but I had to believe it was. With perspiration rolling from my brow and knees that wanted to collapse, I replied, "Give me a minute to get on my clothing." Fear sucked my breath away, but it surged me into motion.

Afraid to leave, but more afraid to stay, I stepped out into the blustery night and hardly touched the ice and snow as I raced to my car. It was midnight. My mind raced. Where should I go? What is he going to do with the gun? Will someone get hurt? Oh God, help us! The short trip to our son, Walter's house seemed 100 miles away, and it took forever to get there. I prayed all the way. By the time I reached his house, I was very excited and had difficulty explaining what was going on.

When he understood, he said, "Let me throw on some clothes, and we'll go see what's happening."

We approached the house with terror, and an imagination filled with all sorts of horrible outcomes. When we went inside, we found Henry in bed and asleep. The gun was on the table.

Grabbing the gun, we reflected on what we had learned by courting disaster. Guns are not safe for us to allow in our home.

Prayer: - Thank you Father, for keeping us safe. I was afraid to come home and see what happened to Henry. I am so grateful that he was safe and no one was harmed.

Going to Walter's house was the perfect answer - this time. Thank you for directing me to go there. It was a blessing that Walter was home, and he knew what to do. That helped to calm me. Thank you for having Henry asleep when we came back. The whole episode was frightening. Thank you for all you have bestowed upon us. Amen

Rapist Moved In

It seemed to be a normal day. Henry was happy with the TV playing in the background. Our daughter was delighted with "her show." It was one of those "Soap Operas" that she thought she couldn't miss.

I had the freedom to get some work done while the TV consumed their attention. I was glad to have Henry focusing on something other than my activities.

After watching the show for a short time, he began to pace. At first I thought he was just restless, but then I looked at his face. He was gritting his teeth and clenching his jaw. He was obviously distressed. A frown appeared on his sweat-glistening brow as he began to mutter in a nearly inaudible tone.

"What was that you said, Henry?"

He was startled by my question. Then, in a whisper he said, "I am looking for the police."

Puzzled, I asked, "Why?"

As if it was the most natural thing to say, he blurted, "They are going to arrest me."

I thought, Now what has he done?

As if he could hear my thoughts, he said, "You know, for the rape I committed."

Now I was speechless. Where would he get such an idea? He surely hasn't been anywhere except with one of us, so how can he form such a thought?

Our daughter drew me to one side and said, "Mom, do you think that Dad took on the identity of the perpetrator of the rape on the TV show? It is hard to comprehend, but I think that's what happened."

Prayer: - Father, this is a tough one. It appears that Henry is unable to tell what is real and what is make-believe.

I thought we had a winning combination when we got him interested in watching TV. It appeared to be the right thing to do. Now that he misperceived what happened, I am filled with the need to protect him from the effects of the TV set.

Engulf me with the thoughts that will keep him safe from the dangers inherent in viewing the TV. I am filled with the thought of re-

stricting his TV viewing. I fight myself with that choice, because when he watches, it gives me a break.

Surround me with thoughts of a better way to work with him. Clear his mind of the worry of the unreal, and grant him peace. Instill in my mind the things that will nurture and assure him. I pray for the best for him. Amen

Section III
Late Stage

Fuzzy Flowers

Everything appears the same; yet nothing is. The flowers are fuzzy, as my tears mingle with the dew.

My heart skips a beat while sorrow is a cloak around me. No one notices! The biggest grief I have ever experienced, but nobody stops! I want to grasp each passerby and say, "Can't you see, the love of my life does not know me?" The world moves on. Death is understood as a part of living, but most people can't comprehend this living death. I want to share my grief, but my most important person does not know me.

Prayer: - Father, today I found how it feels to have the one that I love, denying he knows me. I always hoped that it would never happen to us. I was overwhelmed with emotion. It hurt so much.

I tried to excuse it due to his illness, but the pain remained. Then I thought to focus on you to carry both of us. Thank you for not forgetting us and bringing us strength and comfort. Walk with me too. Amen

Living Tribute

Delivering the eulogy for Anne, my long-time friend, was a privilege. However, I was saddened by the fact that she couldn't experience the words of praise.

After the funeral, the news came to me that Helena--one beautiful lady--was diagnosed with an incurable illness. She was not expected to live long.

While thoughts of Helena filled my mind, Anne's recent funeral became the catalyst for a new idea. At least once in their lifetime, people need to hear the affirming things others think of them.

But should I be the one to tell Helena now what she meant to those around her? Would she accept my living tribute? Would the words I'd write about her be helpful? Or would they only increase her fears of the unknown?

After praying about it, I knew what I had to do: write the living tribute, and then decide what to do with it.

Because she is a marvelous person, my writing task was easy. Helena lived her life acknowledging that she was a child of God-and that she was within His sheltering wings.

After preparing the tribute, I made the decision to share it with Helena, and promptly paid her a visit. I shored up my faith with silent prayers, and drew close to her bedside.

"I've jotted down some thoughts about you," I said hesitatingly. "May I share them with you?" Her affirmative response encouraged and calmed me. Quietly, I read the words I'd written as Helena's living tribute. Her radiant face moved me to tears.

I left Helena feeling that we'd shared some meaningful moments. But only later was I assured of her reaction to my visit. She told a friend, "Hearing my tribute spoken while I am able, is one of the most enriching experiences of my lifetime."

When I think that I almost missed that grand opportunity, I give thanks for God's nudges.

Helena's life was a blessing. Her attitudes and actions were inspirational. She needed to know that someone felt that way about her. And I really needed to tell her.

Then I thought about Henry and the losses he is experiencing.

While he is still able to understand, he also needs affirmation and knowledge of my good feelings about him.

I have found the living tributes to be an opportunity for some quality time with those I love.

Prayer: - Father, thank you for the opportunity to share my love with people who are precious to me. Affirmation along life's way, is a wonderful gift. I feel as if I have been given a second chance and it is very powerful.

Thank you for awakening in me a sensitivity to others. May I be filled with a nurturing spirit. Amen

Guests In The House

Henry was pacing. He was looking for something. Just what that was, had me curious, because it usually meant trouble. "Henry, are you hunting for something?"

He walked up and down the hall, peering into every room. His brow seemed fixed in a permanent, but quizzical frown. "No, I'm just checking."

I waited for a short time, then I asked, "What are you checking?" Then he assumed his mysterious stance. "Something," he whispered softly.

I started talking to myself, "Patience, Carole, keep your patience. He will tell you when he is ready." He seemed puzzled and not in his "take things apart phase." At least, I hoped that was true.

Finally he blurted, "Where are you keeping my brother, Tim?"

Without thinking, my rational response kicked in, "He's not here, he's at his house."

"I know he stays here, I saw him a little while ago."

In an attempt to redirect, "Were you able to talk to him? What was it you talked about? Did he give any indication when he would be coming back?"

Thinking of no other way to sidetrack him, and with a calm I didn't feel, I said, "When he comes, we can pull out the cot, but now I need some help with dinner. Will you help me?"

Together, we trotted off to the kitchen, and started a successful diversionary tactic. When it worked, I uttered a prayer of thanks to God. Henry surely keeps my mind on alert.

Prayer: - Lord, I could use more patience, and my impatience says I want it right now. Henry's illness causes me to think in ways I never did before. I thank you for inspiring that distraction. It worked well today. It's so hard to know what to say and how to react when he's so confused. I know that what works today may not work tomorrow. Fill me with the wisdom to know what to do and say, and fill us with attitudes that will keep the peace. Help me to focus on you. Amen

Greasing My Palm

The sun was shining. My spirit was encouraged with the day's fresh, clean breeze.

The smell of coffee brewing, and the subtle sizzle of eggs frying in the pan restored memories of the time when Henry was well--when the world was ours to conquer.

As I reached for a plate on the shelf, my fingers fell on a glob of butter. Henry was at it again. He had mixed several "yukky" dishes among the clean ones. What a mess!

Why is it that everything I do has to be done twice? Is anyone interested in knowing that lately doing things just once is enough to wear me out?

I catch my breath. "Carole," I said to myself, "focus on what's important. Aren't you thankful that Henry is struggling to help you? Aren't you glad you're still together?"

I sit back, then sip my coffee from a clean cup and utter, "Indeed, I have much for which to be thankful."

Prayer: - Thank you for the beauty of the day, and it's still beautiful, even though I got upset at a glob of butter. Forgive me for struggling with the little things.

Henry tries so hard to help me. There are times when I find it difficult to see that. It's harder when my clean dishes are butter coated. But God, I am trying to see and appreciate all the good in this man I love.

I keep asking for patience, but it seems that I continue to want it right now. Forgive my impatience.

Grant me the strength and courage I need to face all that lies ahead and allow Henry to be encompassed in love. Amen

The Day of Feasting

The day seemed ordinary, but Henry was agitated and restless. There seemed no way to calm him. "Henry, what are you looking for?"

Instantly, he said, "I need a place to put 'em,"

"Put what, Henry?"

"You know."

"No Henry, you tell me."

"Well, all this stuff."

"What stuff?"

"You know. All this food."

Looking around I saw no food, and I had no idea what he was talking about. "Henry, what food?"

"The food is all over the place and we've got to do something or it will spoil," he insisted.

I was still puzzled when, Cheryl, our daughter who sat with him while I ran to the store, came back from her errands. I said, "Maybe you can shed some light on our mystery."

I explained our conversations and asked, "Cheryl, do you have an explanation for his upset?"

She laughed gently as she said, "Mother, we watched a cooking show, and you know how they make all sorts of food. I believe Dad thinks we have all that food here. In his mind, we were really there and part of it."

Now, I understood his dilemma, and that is the first step in finding a solution. Although there was no food, I had to find a way to satisfy Henry that the food would be OK. Finally, I said, "The food is all refrigerated," and Henry was quieted.

Prayer: - Father, it seems that we go from one new adventure to the next. This business of believing the TV to be actual events was not in my thinking.

Thank you for leading us to the help to find the source of his distress. Once we got headed in the right direction, the answer was so simple.

There are times when I need reminders to focus on the good in all that happens. Thank you for all our blessings. It would be helpful if

Henry was more in touch with reality, but I'm grateful that he's able to pay attention to things around him. Help us to maximize his abilities, and to deal more effectively with his disabilities. Amen

Unsolved Mystery

Our youngest was about to be married. Everything seemed to be falling into place. We had the birth certificate from the vault. Now all we had to do was to take it to the courthouse and apply for the marriage license.

When she was about to leave, my daughter called out, "Has anyone seen my birth certificate?"

Rounds of questions flew through the air.

"Where did you last have it?"

"Are you sure you put it there?"

"Where else might you have stashed it?"

"Could you have put it in the car?"

Then, almost simultaneously, we all turned towards Henry.

"Have you seen the birth certificate?" we all asked at once.

"What does it look like?" Henry questioned. Then, he offered, "No, I haven't seen it. Those things are valuable, and you're supposed to take good care of them."

And so the search continued. We looked upstairs, downstairs, over, under, and inside of everything. Finally, we had to admit that the birth certificate was lost.

We rushed our order to Harrisburg for a duplicate, and explained that we had to have it in time for the wedding day.

In the end, it did arrive in time for our daughter's wedding. But it wasn't until five years later--on one of those very ordinary days--that Henry came to me with an extraordinary find.

"You'll never guess what I found in an old magazine," he said. "Look, I found a birth certificate. You know, you should take better care of things like this."

Prayer: - I guess I just had a lesson in patience, God. I think that I would never have found that hiding place, even if we had looked steadily for five years.

Thank you, God, for showing him that secret spot. It is one that would never come to my mind. We marvel that Henry was alert enough to recognize that he had something of signifigance. That was her original birth certificate, so I am very appreciative.

It would be easier if Henry would stop hiding things, but if that is not to be, perhaps you would heighten our skill at finding things.

Strengthen our sense of your presence and still our restlessness. Amen

Sleepy Eyes

Three AM and Henry was finally ready to "rest his eyes" in the prone position in bed. Exhaustion washed over me in waves. I eased myself gently onto the bed and drifted off into a deepening sleep. Even then, I was in what I call my "alert mode." I needed to stay alert to changes in sound or movement, because Henry often wandered away.

My antenna jumped to attention. Something was amiss. Still struggling from lack of sleep, I stretched out in the bed, trying to orient myself from the depths of sleep. My arms reached fully out to the side. Whoops! Suddenly, I absorbed what was wrong. Henry was out of bed again. I knew that I had no choice but to check on what he was doing. I pulled myself to an upright position, and hunted for my glasses to see the time. Although the house was brightly lit, I thought I had just gotten to bed.

Reality finally hit me. It's only 4:00 AM, no wonder I'm tired. As I entered the kitchen area, the bright lights, a poorly tuned radio, the smell of coffee, and a fully dressed mate greeted me. And, I was filled with hope that he was just getting a drink.

With a calm and cheerfulness I did not feel, I asked "Henry, what are you doing?"

He looked me straight in the eye and said, "I'm not like some people around here, I'm getting ready for church on time. I was just going to wake you."

I blurted, "Henry, it's the middle of the night, and today is Tuesday."

Just as quickly he said, "You aren't going to fool me with your silliness, because I know you would really like to sleep."

He was right about the latter. I really wanted to sleep, but it was not to be any more that night. I had to work to convince him not to leave the house. The time of the day, and the day of the week were out of his grasp. I gave thanks that I managed to persuade him to stay home.

Prayer: - Father, I cling to your promise that you will be with me always. If ever I needed you, it's now, during these troubling and exhausting times. I know you know how Henry can sometimes be confused and stubborn, but I want to tell you it's troubling both of us.

I need guidance, and I crave restful sleep. Comfort Henry as he agonizes over getting to the church on time. We both need a touch of calm and patience, and anything else that would help us to function better.

Grant me the ability to know the things that I need to know to keep the peace. Fill us with your calming presence. Amen

Clothing How-To

Henry bounded through the halls with his underpants in his hand and nothing on his body. He held his britches upside down and by the leg. He explained that he was not able to get his feet through that hole, and he pointed sideways. He asked, "Do you know the way to use this underwear?"

He was asking big questions about his other clothing as well. His frightened expression touched me deeply. This was our first venture into loss of memory for this kind of knowledge, and tears wet my eyes. I wanted to draw him close and rock him like a child, but his manner prohibited that. I needed to steady his confusion and assist him in dressing for the day. The simplest garment required a great deal of explanation and maneuvering.

Although his condition was deteriorating, I wasn't ready for this.

I wanted to share with someone else that this was an educated man, and it shouldn't be like this. The emotion within my head shouted that the illness is unfair, then a more rational side responded that illness has nothing to do with fair. Illness just is.

Prayer: - Thank you for the privilege of being able to be there for my love. I appreciate the chance to help and guide him, as he always was able to guide me. Dear heavenly Father, I detest the idea that he needs this kind of support.

Show us the way to comfort him in his increasing dependence. Allow love to shine through it all. We have turned our lives to your care. Use us as you will. Amen

The Dead Man In My Chair

"He's there, sitting in the chair. I saw him myself. I talked to him just a short time ago." Henry was so animated as he told me how his cousin, who was dead for a long time, was there in my living room. Without thought, my logical mind spoke up, "But, Henry, Wilbur has been dead for years." As soon as the words left my mouth, I knew I made a mistake in stating what seemed obvious to me.

Henry reacted in great distress. He shouted, "You mean Wilbur died and no one told me about it? Why would you hide things like that? . . . Anyway, you're wrong. He is alive, because I spoke to him. I saw him myself. . . Don't tell me to calm down. I know what I saw."

Pausing to regroup, I thought, What can I say that would calm the situation? How can I act to ease his agitation? I desperately wanted to convince him that what he saw was in his mind. Early in the course of this illness, I found arguing would cause more trouble.
As if someone spoke, I heard "Change the subject." I tried, but Henry was determined to stay with it.

"You said Wilbur is dead! How can he sit in the chair if he's dead? Why would you be so nasty?"

Back off and give him space, echoed in the crevices of my mind. I retreated.

Henry began to mutter, "She tried to tell me a dead man was sitting in my chair. I know what I saw and Wilbur was not dead."
As time passed, Henry became less agitated in his pacing. I offered him some pie and he seemed calmed. He gave no indication that he remembered our earlier confrontation. This time the loss of memory was working for us. Thank God for that part.

Prayer: - Father, my logical mind is my handicap. When Henry said he saw his cousin, I fought him, because I knew he was dead. Although he knew it before, he's forgotten. Now it's new grief.

Grant me the wisdom to know when it is necessary for Henry to confront the truth and when it isn't. When there is another way, place in my mind the way to do it. We need all the help we can get.

Comfort Henry in his agitation, and I guess I could stand some comforting too. I turn it all over to you. Amen

Memories

Once again a friend uttered those dreaded words, "I don't like to visit him, because I want to remember him the way he was."
Do they really think that will make me understand why they avoid visiting or being with us?

I hold back the pain and anger that thoughtless comment evokes. Inside I shout, "Don't you realize that I want to remember all that he has been, too? Unless some memory impairment intervenes with us, we'll continue to remember him as he has always been, while we must continue to support and affirm him in the way he's become."

Under my breath I said, "You're not supposed to be the one with the memory problem, he is. Take care of him as he is now, and share with him now the good things you remember. There will be plenty of time later to remember who he was."

One of these times, I might verbalize my thoughts.

Prayer: - I didn't spout my anger Father, but forgive me for feeling so strongly. I choose not to get angry, but at times it happens. I love those who make the insensitive remarks, but I want to pour an understanding of Henry into them. When I feel that way, it is hard to show love.

Enable us to communicate our needs to others. Open their eyes and hearts to the situation. Cloak us all in your love and fill us all with compassion. Amen

The "Forever Vow"

Forty years ago, we pledged to God and to each other, "For better or worse." When we joined, we visualized "worse" to be the blending of our differences.

He's a morning person, and I'm a night person. He awakens alert and I don't. He's hot and I'm cold. He works to gain weight, and I try to lose weight. He's tall and I'm short.

Working to smooth the rough times, we discovered that our love for each other is the glue that makes the "worse," better.

When we married, we shared a mattress on the floor until our "specially made tall bed" arrived. We shared our prayers, our love, our hopes and dreams in that bed. We accommodated our differences with some creative planning.

So now what was my problem? We were in the midst of the worst of the "worse". Henry was diagnosed with Alzheimer's disease, and it tilted our universe. Increasingly, Henry's slowed thoughts separated us, and I longed for the man of our youth, or even of months earlier.

Oh, I loved him more, but that didn't stop the pain. He was incapable of communicating in the same ways. It was as if a stranger had come to stay and my sweet thoughtful Henry was not recognizable. Oh, his physical characteristics appeared essentially the same, but older.

One problem was that I was tired. Henry mixed night with day. If I was inattentive as we started to bed, he thought it was time to get up, then he dressed himself, and asked for breakfast. He was up all night.

When he finally settled down I unfolded my weary body at his side, he reached over and pulled the hair on my arm. If I would lie silently, ready to scream, he'd become more aggressive and he made little pinches along my arm. If I'd complain, he became irritated and would say, "I'm just doing a little loving."

But I couldn't sleep while he was doing that. I prayed, "Oh God, why am I so irritable?"

I was very tense until he was asleep. If I didn't move in bed, I had pain, and if I did move, he awakened and the whole procedure began again, or he thought it was time to get up. And whenever he got up, I had to persuade him, especially in the middle of the night, not to call a friend.

Henry had what is called "sun-downing." At sunset he became very active. Then, he had more energy than ten people did.

He napped during the day, but I couldn't prevent that. When he sat down he rested. I roused him in the daytime and increased his exercise so that he would sleep at night, but it didn't work.

He was a bundle of energy. It was hard for me to last the day. I loved him deeply, but I needed rest. My heart screamed, "Please give me about six days of uninterrupted sleep, blissful rest."

Now, torn by guilt, I thought the impossible. After forty years, I considered moving out of our bed to another room, away from my husband.

I prayed, "Oh God, how can I think of it? Father, forgive me. I don't know what to do. I can't sleep. I've been sick. I'm irritable. I don't like myself for thinking this, let alone doing it. In fact, I hate 'me' for thinking of this option. I promised 'for better or worse,' and now I'm leaving his bed while he fights his fears through the 'worse.' I'm not very nice, because I can't fight this 'worse.' God, I'm so mixed up. I want to do what's right, but nothing seems right. I don't want to hurt him, and I know if I leave our bed, it will hurt. My head and my heart argue. Guide me in thinking this through."

"I know the answer isn't easy. It's difficult to discuss the conflict with anyone because it's so personal and filled with my beliefs about you and our absolute loyalty of marriage. I don't want to be confused by someone who does not hold my beliefs, because I'm already torn apart trying to find a solution."

"God, I know what I have to do, but I don't want to do this. It seems so wrong. I want to feel his caress and body next to mine. I love him so much. I'm going to go under if I can't get any sleep. God help him to understand. Comfort us. Please show me if there's another way."

As I moved my things into the spare bedroom, tears flowed down my cheeks. God, I'm not ready to deal with Henry. But he won't wait.

He pleaded: "What do you mean you're going to sleep there?

What did I do? Why are you mad at me? Don't you love me anymore? How could you do this? Did you find someone else? You can't leave me."

My resolve weakened, but I knew that I couldn't help him if I was sick, and I would get sick if I didn't get my rest.

I reached for Henry and we embraced. "I love you more than ever. I'm doing this for both of us. Henry, let's pray about this."

I grasped his hand and we prayed, "God, help us to feel your love and then to feel each other's love. We're both hurting. Please comfort us. Allow us to follow your will and way. We are yours first. Help us to adjust to this change and grant us peace. Amen"

We were both heartbroken, but became more accepting. Within a few days the loss of memory worked for us. Henry didn't remember. He was usually contented with the arrangement. I accepted it because it was the right thing for both of us, but I still grieved.

I learned that God will help us through the "better or worse," but only on His terms.

Prayer: - Father, I still need the assurance that I didn't abandon Henry and that I made it possible to be available through the "worse." I know I did what I had to do to save both of us, but I have difficulty finding peace with that. I am thankful for the closeness we still share. Amen

Who's Calling?

Some time ago, Henry started to become confused by the telephone. He was easy prey to telephone solicitors. On one occasion, I was called first, and said, "No, I don't want any."

They called back and got Henry, and I unwillingly had to pay $100.00 for what I had refused to buy, and he accepted.

With the loss of some of my hearing, I couldn't always hear the telephone when it rang. Henry could not remember to "not answer" the phone, or to come tell me it was ringing. I got an answering machine to help, but he would answer it before I was aware it rang and without allowing the new machine to respond.

Henry developed new abilities to accommodate this different turn of events. He became a silent sprinter. He could catch the phone on one ring, no matter where he was.

He took messages, which became partial or nonexistent by the time I heard about them. He had no memory about who called or what they wanted, and he bought and committed to all sorts of things.

I could find nothing that worked, and I tried louder bells and flashing lights, and the machine, but he could still catch it on the first ring, and he would not permit the answering machine solution.

Once, while I was by his side he said, "No, Carole is out and can't be reached."

I begged, "Henry, please let me talk."

He became agitated, pushed me aside, and said, "This is my friend and I am going to talk."

When he was combative, I knew there was no reasoning with him. I never did find out what the call was all about. Through it all, he was trying to help me, but I was still in a communication crisis.

I constantly educated family and friends about the message status, warning them that if I did not return a call, to get back to me. And I prayed for understanding.

As time moved along, Henry didn't run to answer as fast, and people, including Henry, became more used to dealing with a machine first.

Prayer: - God, when I talk to you, I always seem to have some dilemma to think through.

Thank you for being there for all of us, and helping me with the problem solving. The times when it takes longer, I get frustrated and impatient. Show me the places to go and the things to do, to sow peace, and work at my optimum.

Comfort each of us and allow your love to fill every part of our being. We give you all praise and glory. Amen

How Long, Oh God

As I kiss my Henry goodnight, God, I ask you how long do we have to walk hand in hand, each one rejoicing in the other's company? How long do we have left to share the joy of fresh cleansing rain or the newly fallen snow? How long will Henry know the love we have shared?

Will he forget that we married, or who I am? How much time does he have to speak the words of his heart or the thoughts of his mind? How long do we have, God? Will he remember the love magnified in our children? Will he remember you are there, God? How long God, how long?

Prayer: - I ask you how long we have together to do the things we love to share on earth. Forgive me for questioning.

I want you to know that together, in faith, we placed ourselves within your will and way. It is difficult to find that there are some things we can not change and that they require that we trust you completely.

Please stay with us and allow us the awareness that you are there, and through that, we will be together in spirit. Amen

Section IV
Nursing Home

Boundless Love Can't Always Stop Loneliness

"If you loved me you wouldn't do this."

His angry words echoed through my head. Could I have done otherwise? Did I try hard enough?

I love him so much. I would never hurt him, but he is hurting, and so am I. Oh, how I failed him!

I had to make a decision I didn't want to make. In fact, I often said that I never would allow such a thing to happen. Now, because the doctors told me I had to, I placed him in a nursing home.

My feelings are so confusing. I keep echoing that I had no choice at all, but did I? I don't know. Did I try hard enough? Could I have been more patient? Could I have done things differently? Was there another route that I did not explore?

Am I really the selfish person he said that I am? A part of me would affirm his accusations, and that's what makes it so hard. I feel guilty, nasty and mean, because I was sure that this would never be an option.

It is understandable that I'm unable to convince him that I could do nothing else, because I can't accept this change myself. My heart has been broken in two. As my tears wet the pillow, I struggle to find a way for him to see my love.

How can he understand that it is because of that love, and that I want the strength to be there for him, that he must leave his home of 40 years? He can't remember who I am, so why do I torture myself with unrealistic expectations? I pray for the miracle of acceptance.

But the house shouts in its silence. His empty chair is begging for the warmth of his being. I miss him. I want to look over and see him where he belongs, by my side, but that can't be. I want to share those special moments and talk the way we did before he got sick.

His need for more care than I am physically able to give doesn't lessen my desire to have him home sharing with me. I feel devastated, because he is not here.

His angry words cut a deep groove in my spirit, yet I am unable to change the way it is. My anger is not directed at him, but at the illness, which robs the two of us of our ability to remain together in our home and caring for each other.

Somehow I feel as if I have failed him, yet intellectually, I know that there were no workable options. My heart has trouble accepting that this is true. I want it to be different.

My insecurities are affirmed when my friends say things like, "I didn't know that he was that bad," or "Why would you do something like that?" I question my choices and I hurt even more. I choose not to burden my children.

I can't share with my husband, and my friends' remarks indicate that they don't understand. The sense of being utterly alone to face the world causes my feelings to intensify.

As I search for help and understanding, will someone be there for me? I won't know unless somebody reaches out to me.

Prayer: - Oh my dear God, I have searched for ways to make another choice, because I didn't want to come to this conclusion. This was one of the hardest things I had to do. Give me strength.

My head knows he is where he should be, but my heart struggles to allow him to stay there. Anything short of being together fills me with sorrow.

Help us both to make the adjustment, and find peace. Amen

The Seeker

His knobby fingers work the edges of his hanky as he paces the hall. His lean, lanky frame moves like an old agitator washer, up and down as he sways sideways.

His cane tap-tap-taps as he searches. Now he seeks the train station, yesterday it was his brother, and nobody knows what tomorrow will bring.

Ever pursuing a way back by my side, he tries the locks on all the doors. None are working for him. His objective delayed, he is drawn by the music in the common room. There is momentary calm as he enters and then "sings along."

Prayer: - It is difficult to watch him always seeking, often seeking what can't be. I rejoice that he still has music to comfort him. He always loved to sing, and I am grateful for every opportunity that he has to participate.

Thank you for the time that we are able to spend together, particularly when he has awareness of me and of our surroundings.

You have patiently taught me to appreciate the little triumphs. I ever seek an awareness of them.

Please watch over each of us, when we are apart. Amen

Conversations: Good News - Bad News

Carole, I was sorry to learn Henry was admitted to a Nursing Home.

The good news is that a suitable place was available.

But it's so sad to see someone with such a great mind doing the activities associated with a child.

Friend, the good news is that he finds pleasure in such activities.

Carole, don't you understand? They were singing children's songs!

Ah, yes. It's great that he can remember them, and finds joy in singing the happy songs, and the hymns of our faith!

Can't you see that sometimes he's agitated?

Yes, that's true, but they work as a team to distract and comfort him. I was exhausted working alone.

He's so slow and plays with his food when he eats.

But I am so glad he's able to eat.

It must be hard to see him wear outfits that don't match.

I am happy that his clothing is clean and dry, and that he is content with wearing clothes, because it was not always so.

But, he told me his brother was there with him, and you know he isn't!

Isn't it great that when his brother can't be with him, he's able to find comfort in those who are around him?

Doesn't it bother you that at times he thinks you're someone else?

Yes, but it helps when he finds me to be someone he cares for, and someone who is important in his life.

He told me his mother just died. How are you managing the funeral?

His mother died twenty years ago, so we work to talk through trips into the happier times when she was alive. We are relieved when that distraction works.

Doesn't it bother you that you're separated from him?

Of course, but by getting rest, I'm more available than before.

Carole, I'm uncomfortable visiting him.

When you visit him you nurture me. Sometimes you break through his confusion.

I never know what to say.

The important thing about what you say is that you speak in love and avoid arguments.

I just want to remember him as he was!

Dealing with who he is now doesn't erase the way he was, but it does nourish who he has become.

When I see him I want to cry.

Tears are an honest reaction and show great feeling. Even Jesus wept. I am thankful for friends who care. It eases my sorrow to know you care. Thank you for walking with me today.

Prayer: - Father, thank you for friends who are willing to share their true feelings, and then are willing to allow me to share my reactions to their comments. It helps me to feel more freedom of true communication.

Bless those who care enough to express themselves in such a way.

Empower us all to be the best that we can be, and sensitize us to the feelings of others. Amen

The Repairman

Henry is with Wilbur, a fellow resident. They're "working" on an up-ended bedside table. Heads together, they whisper to each other as Henry spins the wheels, and Wilbur is moving the table first up, then down ... up and down.

They're happy. They're "fixing" something. They return the table to its upright position, at last. They wipe their hands and exclaim to each other, "It's fixed!"

But Henry keeps moving. I watch as he pulls the drawers of the dresser in, then out ... out and in... in and out. When he notices me, he lets me know, "I had a lot of work to do today, but I got only part of it done. I'll have to keep working, if we're going to make time to talk."

Prayer: - Did you notice how content Henry is when he finds something he can fix, Father? I am thankful that he can be busy, and find something that satisfies him. It's so helpful to have him in a protected environment and away from any heavy-duty destructive-take-things-apart place. The staff, where he is, has more than one pair of eyes to watch him. I thank you that they allow him to work on things and act lovingly with him.

Continue to strengthen those who care for him and keep Henry in your protection. Guide each of us, and grant us rest. Amen

The Architect

He's working as though he's the designer of the most complicated architectural drawing. I'm watching Henry and my mind is reeling. I see him place the last piece in the pre-school puzzle. He shows his "masterpiece" to anyone he can find, and a smile born of pride wreathes his face.

"Where is the Henry I married forty years ago?" My heart screams, "Where is my Master of Design--the man I knew--my Henry with the brilliant mind and engaging conversation?"

My husband's dancing eyes always reflected his joy of living. Now when I look at Henry, I see only a glimmer of that sparkle ... and then it's filtered through my tears.

What a marvelous storyteller Henry was! The stories he wants to tell me now, are of times long passed.

When I try to discuss with him the things we've shared, I watch how his mind struggles to grasp for fleeting pieces of memory. But to Henry, our history is new information. Even so, it delights him. On those rare occasions when Henry is able to identify events, he's overjoyed.

"I remember some of that," he'll say. I love the way those words roll happily from his tongue. That tiny bit of memory lights up his face--he's like a child receiving a new toy.

Someone has pulled another pre-school puzzle from the closet. Henry's about to build another masterpiece.

Prayer: - Although I'm pleased that Henry is content, I also feel sad that such simple things are all he's able to master. I give thanks that he still can find pleasure, but I am bothered by his child-like delights. Reform my ideas about the simplicity of what he enjoys.

Provide opportunity for him to operate in the most positive ways, and lead me in ways of accepting and affirming him, right where he is. Amen

Seatmates

This is another one of those days when Henry can't identify people correctly. At times he longs for visits from people we've known for years. I notice that he's particularly homesick for people of our church group who are longtime friends. It has been one year since we were together with the group at our summer rental cottage, and there prepared a meal for them.

I don't know how long Henry will be able to recognize our friends. While he still is able to enjoy sharing memories, I feel an urgency to do something positive to enhance his pleasure. My first inclination is to plan a dinner at the nursing home, but I am unsure if that can happen.

After making some arrangements, I asked the group from our church to the party. They agreed to come and offered to lessen my costs by paying for their own meals.

I invited a multi-talented, Activities Director from the nursing home to come as a guest and also play the keyboard and sing a duet with Henry. I felt her presence would make it easier for Henry.

When the big night arrived, Henry was happy and excited. He joyfully greeted the people. Then when the food arrived, we took our seats at the tables.

Henry and I sat together and looked for others to join us. But one by one, our classmates found their places at other tables. "Won't you come and join us?" I asked first one couple, and then another. But no one would sit with us. One person was about to do so, but then looked around and said, "I want to sit with my friends."

Of course I was hurt. The pain within me increased as I thought who is this party to benefit? In the end, latecomers joined us, and that eased my discomfort.

To enjoy Henry's party, I had to focus some of my attention to blotting out the unintentional pain. The phrase, "They knew not what they did," filled my thoughts. I focused on excusing and moving on. Nobody else seemed to be aware that his or her behavior could be perceived as hurtful.

As the evening progressed, Henry told stories of yesteryear as though they were happening today. And the people who heard the tales asked me questions as though they also thought he was relating current events. I wanted to blurt out, "Don't you realize, he is confused and talking of events of years gone by as though they just happened?"

I had to put that aside as I focused on the fact that Henry was delighted with the party. Therefore, I concluded that the evening was a success. Henry was happy, and overall, we had a fun-filled evening.

Prayer: - God, here I am again, with a problem. I know we have had so many blessings, but tonight we had a gathering of friends.

I'm ashamed to say I was troubled when we waited so long for somebody to come to sit with us. When folks believed he was better than he really was, I was upset and felt angry. Forgive me.

I need help with my feelings and reactions. Maybe you would help me to find a way to let people know how this felt, so that it won't happen to someone else.

As I think about it, at some time I may have been guilty of this kind of thoughtlessness.

God, open our eyes that we might see how we act as others do. Temper our words and actions with compassion.

Take this burden from me and show me the way to rejoice in all things. Amen

Tricks of the Trade

I had to learn behavior basics. Keeping records of actions and conversations immediately preceding behavioral problems has been my best tool in averting the actions in the future. Making an accurate assessment of conversations of those around Henry, when the problem develops, provides essential clues for preventing trouble in the future.

When I said, "Henry, you must take a bath right away," it sounded as if I was attacking, or in a parenting mode. I discovered that when Henry or other adults feel they are losing control of their lives, a commanding attitude becomes threatening to them.

I found a better way. I said, "Henry, would you rather have your bath at 7:00 PM or 9:00 PM?" Then I asked Henry to make a note about the time. I occupied him with other things until the selected time came.

When the time arrived, I said, "Henry, I see your note here." When he acknowledged, I said, "I guess you wanted a bath now, would you like some help?"

I discovered that by offering a choice of workable options, I averted trouble.

Then, I also have to remember; If my first attempt doesn't work, I must reconsider how I handled the whole situation, and try again in a different way.

Prayer: - God, you have promised that your strength is sufficient for all my needs. I have found that some things upset Henry. Open my eyes to see them as they develop. When Henry becomes so agitated, I implore you to give me strength.

Teach me to be more aware of what causes problems, and help me to find the ways to avoid them.

It's in these times of difficulty, that I need your help to remember to lift my praise to you. Thank you God. Amen

The Other Woman

They look like the perfect couple, walking down the hall, each hanging on to the hand of the other. They're happily engrossed in conversation! It's a language known only to them.

Who are they? Why should I care? Shouldn't I be glad to see a senior couple happy? The last answer is yes, but I would rather that he wasn't quite so happy. They are two residents of a dementia unit in a nursing home. He is my long, faithful husband of forty years. He doesn't know who I am. Today I am his mother, yesterday I was his brother, and the day before I became his grandmother. When he starts out, I am never quite sure who he thinks I am.

When he was well, he would not consider holding the hand of another woman. I have to keep reminding myself that this is true. However, knowing that doesn't erase the pain in my heart, it only makes it endurable.

Correcting his misperceptions only angers him. I seek to be with him, but he only wants her company. She gets upset at my attention to him. Today they are possessive of each other. Tomorrow it may be another liaison. Our family has struggled to accept and understand this new range of emotions.

We are forced to face certain basics, and we don't like it. Henry is very confused. In that confusion, he's doing and saying things born of his illness. Imagination and quick thinking are some of the tools we have to use to return him to reality. We have to remain calm and work in a loving, supporting way, but that's easier said than done.

We seem to have many false starts. Then we try something else. Some days it works, but when it doesn't, we work to express our love and hide our pain. Prayer is our companion. Somehow, we move along.

Prayer: - Father, you know the love we shared. At times it's difficult to remember that you are in charge of our lives. Teach us how to deal with this changed Henry. Help me to change what I need to change, and accept those things that are out of my control. Help me to find the support I so deeply feel that I need.

Thank you for the assurance that you will never leave us. Strengthen the sense of your presence. Free us both to be our best. Amen

Second Chance

It has been several weeks now that Henry has forgotten that we are married. A visitor passed by and asked Henry, "Who is your girlfriend?"

He looked me over from head to toe and slowly pronounced, "That's not my girlfriend!"

With a smile she said, "Oh, who is it?"

Frowning and looking deep in thought, he finally said, "She's my mother."

Henry turned and said to me, "I'd like to have a girlfriend, but I don't know how to get one." This continued for several weeks.

The time of our anniversary was fast approaching. I spoke to the Activities Director saying, "It's our anniversary on Wednesday. Henry doesn't know it, but I do. I know he knows and loves a party and ice cream. To celebrate our anniversary we can have ice cream for him and I will know it's for us and our union."

The surprise was mine. When I arrived at the nursing home on "our day," he was talking to me and he looked in my eyes and said, "Will you marry me?'

I was speechless, but after a moment to regroup myself, I said, "Yes."

With a startled and incredulous tone he answered, "You will?"

I said, "I'll go make arrangements."

I went to staff to figure a way to make it happen before he forgot that he proposed. The Chaplain was contacted and it was decided we would do it right after lunch. After lunch I sat by his side and was struck with the thought that he might not remember about the marriage. Thinking that I needed to find out before he was put in an awkward place of choice I stated, "We are getting married shortly."

Instantly he said, "We are?"

Now I was stuck with interpreting that "We are?" Was it good or bad for him? I wasn't sure, so when the chaplain arrived, I told him that the service could not be very long because Henry was unpredictable.

When Henry was asked, "Will you take this woman to be your wife," he shouted a booming, "I do!"

We created a memory, and once again he became the "young buck" that I had married years before. And there in the nursing home we had a wedding reception instead of an anniversary party and we both knew we were married to each other. He chose me again. I have been given a great gift!

Prayer: - Father, this day became filled with a most unexpected pleasure. I started out feeling happy about our anniversary and the party, but sadness that Henry would not know it was our day.

Everything changed when Henry proposed. I was delighted that he asked me, and he was thinking of me as the Carole that he wanted to marry. In some ways our second marriage was just as exciting as the first.

You found a way for us to celebrate that was beyond anything I could imagine. Thank you for such wonderful timing. For all your gifts, we give thanks. Amen

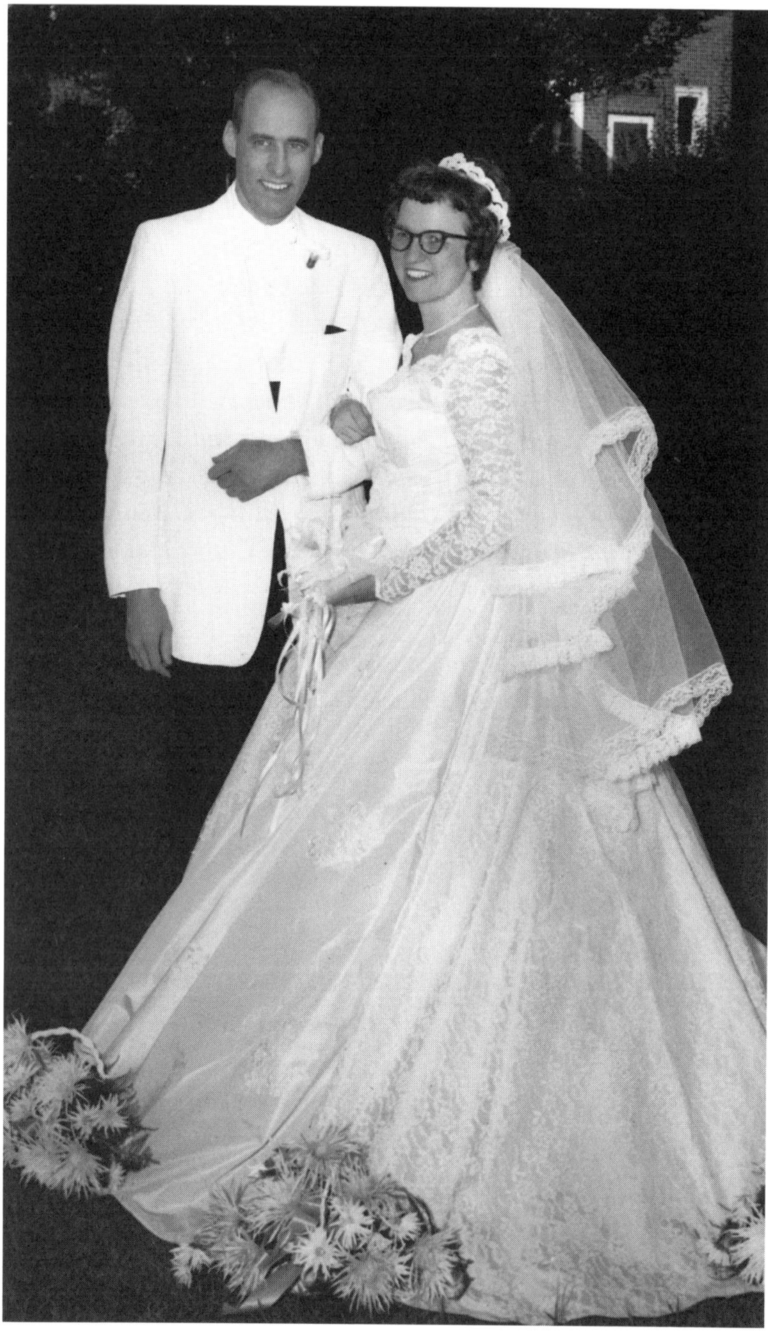

Frank and Carole's First Wedding, September 19, 1959

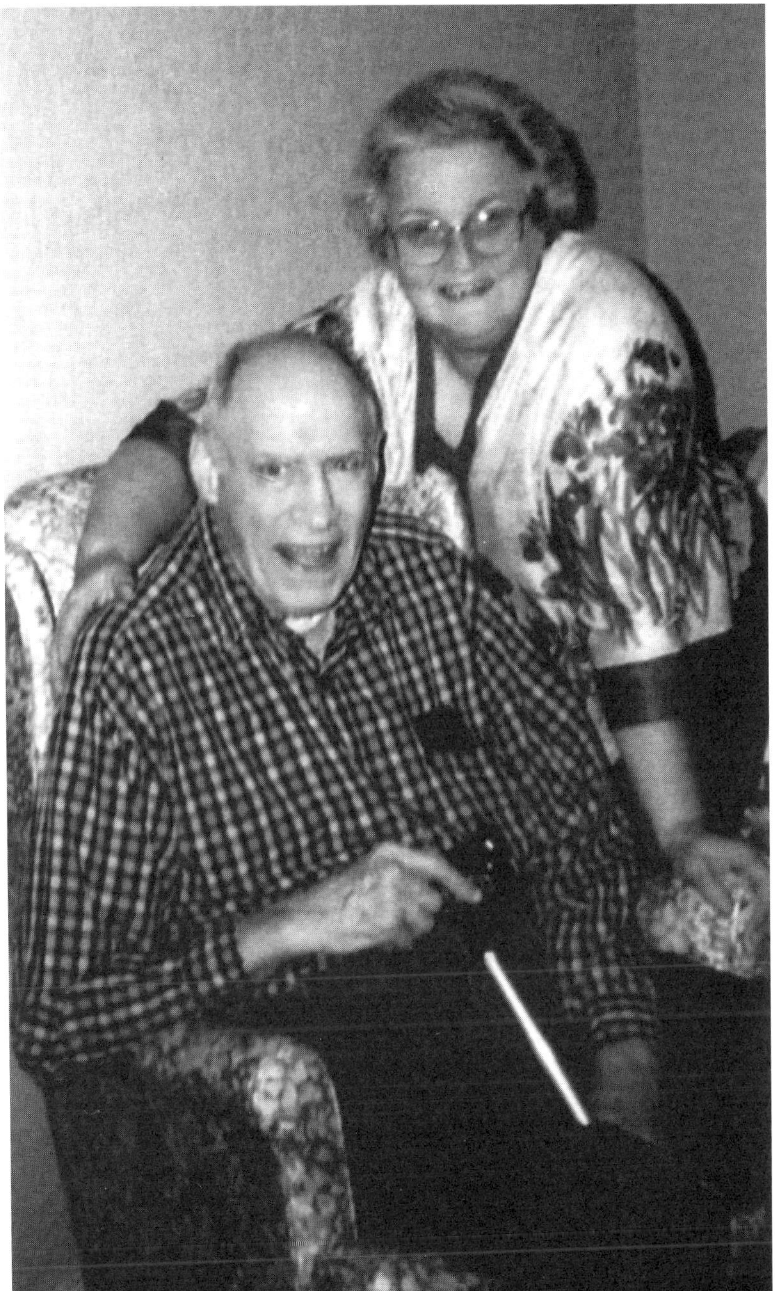

Our Second Wedding, September 19, 2000

Music Nourishes The Spirit

I found that music affects an individual's mood. It may be calming or irritating. Henry and the other dementia patients often were very reactive to music. I found it imperative to choose carefully when picking what they would hear. If they had a religious background, hymns and Gospel choruses were easily remembered, even when all else was forgotten. Yes, the familiar comforted.

"Easy listening" soothes many. As a rule, I aim for the type of music my Henry enjoyed while he was in good health.

Participation in music is a fun thing for Henry and many seniors, or impaired individuals. That includes dance, singing, and/or rhythm type bands. Musical activities are appropriate for a one-on-one set-up or large groups.

In the beginning, I made instruments from things found in most ordinary households:

Butter tubs with a dowel handle, and dry corn or beans inside.

Spoons to clang together, or other objects for a different sound. Pan lids to bang together or tap.

Bells of any kind.

Glasses or empty boxes. (The glasses make different sounds when filled with varying amounts of water. They may be tapped or rubbed around the top with a moistened finger.)

Later, in the nursing home, we used relatively inexpensive rhythm instruments. They are not essential, because the residents may have a good time with any type of instrument, as long as the attitude is happy.

It didn't matter if I chose a sing-along, dance or rhythm band. The most important thing I found is to try something, make it fun, see what works best, and be flexible. Then, I enjoy the experience with them.

Prayer: - Father, you know that I am not a very musical person, but Henry loves it. I enjoy the music, but I am not musically talented. Help me to get over my own reluctance to do musical projects. Remind me that Henry is the benefactor.

When we sing I am reminded to "Make a joyful noise unto the Lord." I wish I made less noise and more music.

Place in our hearts the willingness to create and do different activities.

Thank you for the opportunity to share this activity, because it makes everyone feel better. Amen

Steps to Joy

It was time to make a new beginning. I wanted to put joy into special events and holidays. Graduations and weddings are prime examples of new starts. Either may place strains on our family, or any family affected by dementia.

I soon learned that part of keeping the joy in a happy occasion is preparation. One of the first steps is a reality check. I include such questions as:

"How impaired is my Henry, or loved one?"

"Is he able to be in crowds, or do I need to take precautions?"

"Can I find a way to control the crowds, or sidestep them, if necessary?"

"For the comfort of all, do I need to make special arrangements for the time of the actual event?"

"If I opt to take him in a crowd, should I have an emergency plan for hyperactivity? (That might include someone to stay right with Henry while I am occupied.)"

I must realize that crowds can be overwhelming and demanding, and ask, "Do I need to give consideration to protecting him from the stimulation of the main event?"

If he is unable to take part in the actual event ask, "Is there a way to divide the group and approach him a few at a time?"

"Is there an activity that I may incorporate into the event that Henry may be able to do? i.e. dancing, singing, eating, or visiting etc."

"Am I responding to our own best interests instead of what others might think?"

"Have I considered the timing of the event in relation to his behavior patterns?" (I try to avoid the times that he is more likely to be restless.)

"Can I control the timing if I wanted to do so?"

"If eating is to be part of the day's activities, do I need to make special arrangements to keep Henry safe?"

"Have I taken steps to avoid inappropriate behavior, and do I need to try to prevent overreacting if that occurs?"

"Would it be appropriate to do a 'dry run' with something less structured, or attend an event of lesser importance before the big day?"

My last step is to enjoy the fruits of my preparations. Let the joy of the occasion rule the day.

Prayer: - Thank you for the joy in our lives. Sometimes, we are so busy getting through the day that we forget to seize the things that would bring us pleasure. Sometimes, I seek pleasure and forget to appreciate what I have.

You, oh God, have planted in my heart the fact that I can choose to have a joyful spirit. Bolster me in that choice. Open my mind to the wonders that are mine.

I rejoice in your presence. Amen

Tumult O'er The Fog

My long-time husband is no longer here.
To friends, that statement is not so clear.
He's gone - the one who interacts with me.
It's just his body that they can see.

He once knew everything under the sun.
When he didn't, I sensed trouble had begun.
Soon his daily work he no longer knew,
And he would have to ask me what to do.

He began to have problems finding his way
O'er paths he traveled day after day.
His bright dancing eyes are gone for now.
They have been obscured by a troubled brow.

Simple things stumped him, like figuring math,
Then routine chores like taking a bath.
The basic parts of his own daily care
Became heavy burdens for us to share.

When it came to safely driving the car,
Other's rights exceeded his own by far.
The policeman found he went way too slow;
For safety's sake, his driving had to go.

He'd lost the logic to see it that way.
"My driving is as good as ever," he'd say.
His right to drive seemed the sense of the man.
"Relieved" is the word for the entire clan.

The loss of the loved one who used to be,
Brings sorrow and pain to the family.
Frustration and anger instead of grace
--another person has taken his place.

Our names, our faces, familiar places,
Might as well be in the outer spaces,
Because friends and family he doesn't know,
Although some days it doesn't show.

As time passes there is no way to hide
The troubled confusion that's deep inside.
I work to accept his dependency.
Life has changed for my husband and me.

Prayer: - Dear God, this disease has led us through an obstacle-strewn path. Our emotions rise to the surface. We have learned to work through the difficulties by reaching out to you, but life has definitely changed for all who are near him.

It is so difficult to maximize the blessings that are ours, but give us the wisdom and strength to do that.

We worship you and give you the praise for all our blessings. Amen

Don't We Feel Good?

She said, "We are going to take a bath!"
We never did anything, certainly not take a bath.
I don't even know who she is.
Why does she worry about what I do?

She told me to take my clothes off.
Who does she think I am?
She wanted me to be naked.
I told her I don't do that.

She told me I had to, because I smelled.
I couldn't smell anything.
And, she forgot I took a bath before.
I didn't do anything to get dirty.

She is a bossy little lady.
I sat in the box, without my clothes.
She poured water in there with me.
Then she said, "Watch."

I didn't know what to watch,
I looked all around, for all I could see.
There was just the water and me.
And, the water was wet.

She said, "Scrub with the rag."
I rubbed the sides of the white box.
She got all excited,
"That's not what I meant."

You can't make her happy.
"Fill the rag with some soap,"
Whatever is that?
Besides, where could I fill it?

She took the rag and scrubbed the slippery stuff.
She rubbed my skin with the rag.
I was supposed to rub white bubbles on my skin.
She said, "Now, that's a bath."

She's a funny little lady.
My clothes had been taken away.
She gave me somebody's clothing.
"Wear them," I heard her exclaim.

"Our bath is finished.
Don't we feel good?"
I answered as quickly as I could.
NO!

Prayer: - Father, today I recorded how Henry hears the things we say to him. Thank you for the insight into his thoughts, misperceptions, feelings and then reminding me how easily I am able to annoy him, or confuse him with my conversations.

Help me to speak so that he understands what I mean and allow me to hear what he means.

I needed the bits of humor to better understand gaps in communication..

Enhance our communication skills.

Thank you for being with us to guide and direct all of us. We praise you. Amen

Disease Information

Dementia is an umbrella term for several symptoms related to a decline in thinking skills. Common symptoms include a gradual loss of memory, problems with reasoning or judgment, disorientation, difficulty in learning, loss of language skills, and decline in the ability to perform routine tasks.

People with dementia also experience changes in their personalities and behavioral problems, such as agitation, anxiety, delusions (believing in a reality that does not exist), and hallucinations (seeing things that do not exist).

Alzheimer's *(AHLZ-high-merz)* **disease** is a progressive brain disorder that gradually destroys a person's memory and ability to learn, reason, make judgments, communicate and carry out daily activities. As Alzheimer's progresses, individuals may also experience changes in personality and behavior, such as anxiety, suspiciousness or agitation, as well as delusions or hallucinations.

In late stages of the disease, individuals need help with dressing, personal hygiene, eating and other basic functions. People with Alzheimer's die an average of eight years after first experiencing symptoms, but the duration of the disease can vary from three to 20 years.

Alzheimer's disease is the leading cause of dementia, a group of conditions that all gradually destroy brain cells and leads to progressive decline in mental function. Vascular dementia, another common form, results from reduced blood flow to the brain's nerve cells. In some cases, Alzheimer's disease and vascular dementia can occur together in a condition called "mixed dementia." Other causes of dementia include frontotemporal dementia, dementia with Lewy bodies, Creutzfeldt-Jakob disease and Parkinson's disease.

Diagnosing Alzheimer's disease

Although Alzheimer symptoms can vary widely, the first problem that many people notice is forgetfulness severe enough to affect performance at home, at work or in favorite activities. Other common symptoms include confusion, getting lost in familiar places and difficulty with language. The Alzheimer's Association encourages everyone who notices these symptoms in themselves or someone close to them to consult a physician to obtain a diagnostic assessment.

One important goal of the diagnostic workup is to determine whether symptoms may be due to a condition other than dementia. Depression, medication side effects, certain thyroid conditions, excess use of alcohol and nutritional imbalances are all potentially treatable disorders that may sometimes impair memory or other mental functions. Even if the diagnosis is dementia, timely identification enables individuals to take an active role in treatment decisions and planning for the future.

Disease Information provided by the Alzheimer's Association - Used with permission.

For Information about Alzheimer's disease and dementia or to find the nearest Alzheimer's Support Group contact the Alzheimer's Association at

http://www.alz.org

24/7 Helpline

Contact us for information, referral and support.
tel: 1.800.272.3900
tdd: 1.866.403.3073
e-mail: info@alz.org

National office

225 N. Michigan Ave., Fl. 17
Chicago, IL 60601-7633
tel: 312.335.8700
tdd: 312.335.5886
fax: 1.866.699.1246